The Power of Fasting

How Intermittent Fasting Can Transform Your Life

Lose Weight, Gain Energy, and Develop Complete Mental Clarity

Graham Hodson

The Power of Fasting
How Intermittent Fasting Can Transform Your Life

© Graham Hodson All Rights Reserved 2023

The moral right of the author has been asserted
First published by Rockwood Publishing 2023

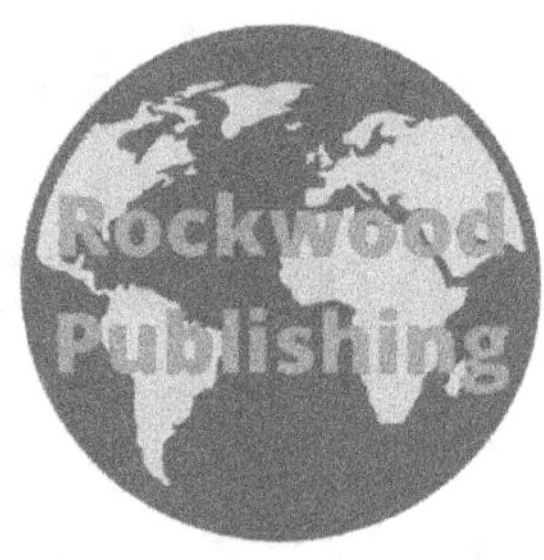

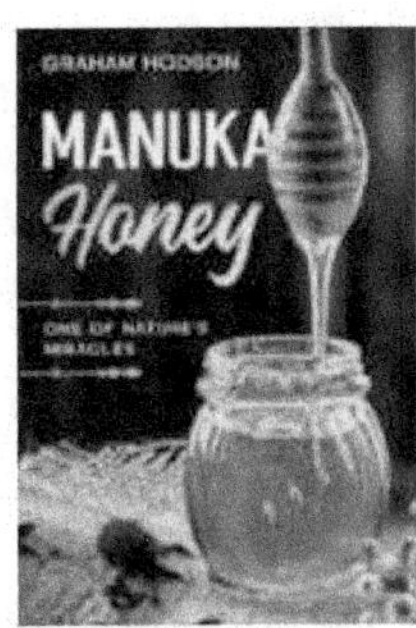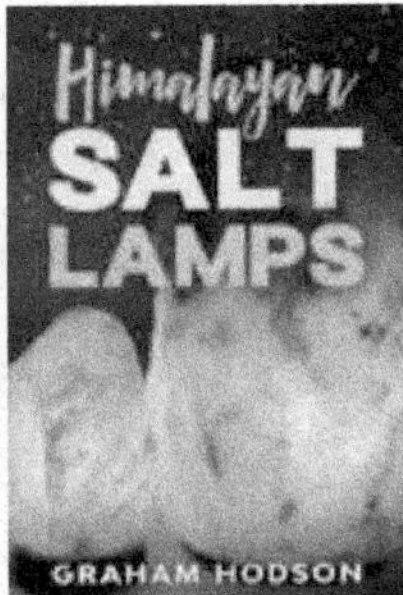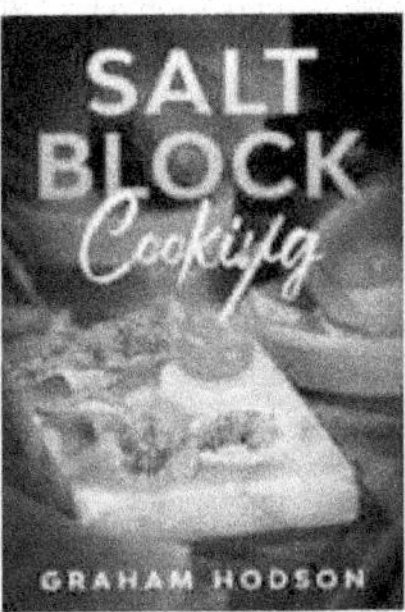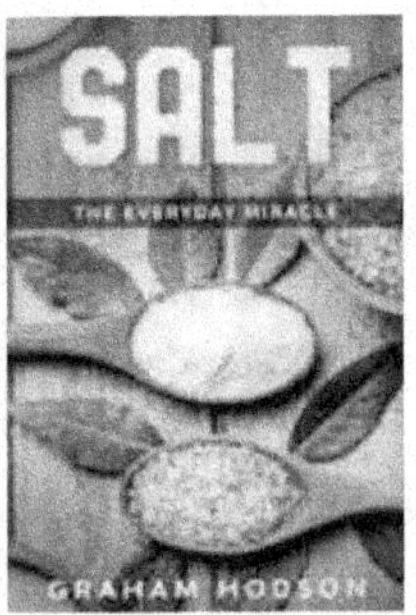
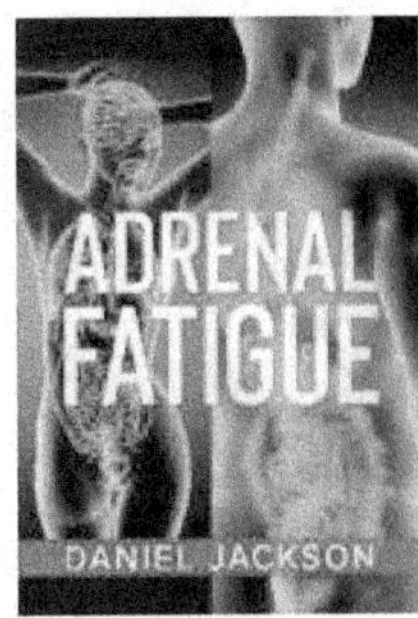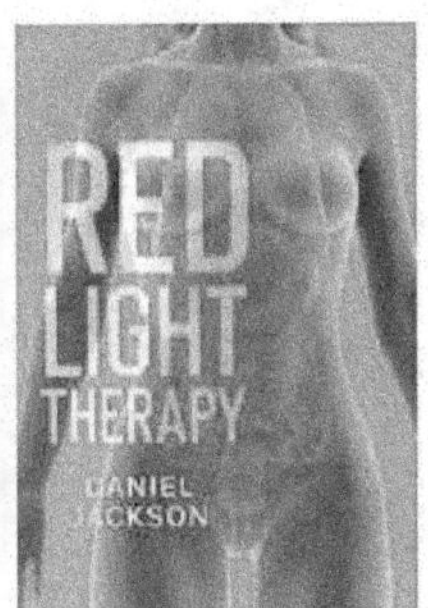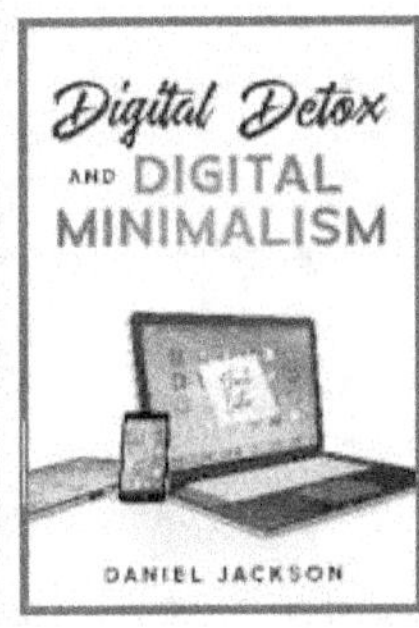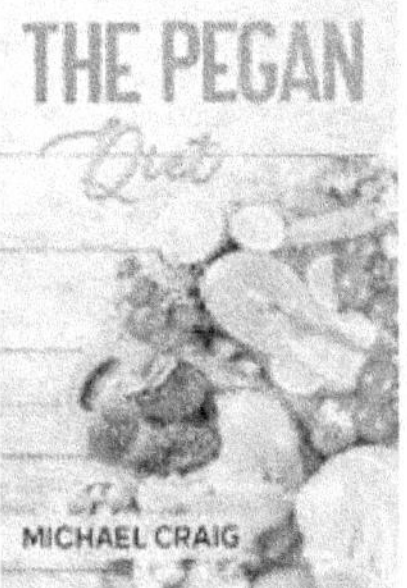

Take a look at more great books available from
Rockwood Publishing

… some for FREE!

Just visit the link below:

rockwoodpublishing.co.uk

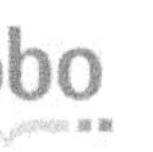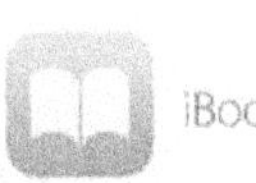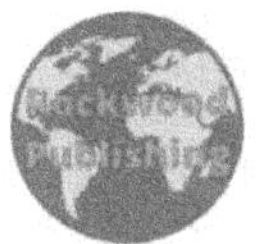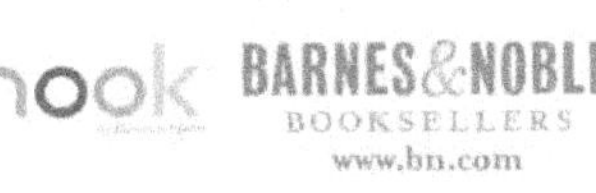

Contents

Chapter 1: Introduction to Intermittent Fasting

The History and Evolution of Fasting

Fasting has been an integral part of human existence for thousands of years. While it may seem like a modern-day fad, the practice has deep roots in our history and has evolved alongside human civilization. In this chapter, we will explore the origins of fasting and how it has developed into the intermittent fasting practices we know today.

The early days of fasting can be traced back to our hunter-gatherer ancestors. Food scarcity was a reality for them, and they would often go through periods of feast and famine. During times of abundance, they would consume large amounts of food, storing excess energy as body fat. This would help them survive during periods of scarcity when food was not readily available. In this sense, fasting was not a voluntary act but a necessary adaptation to an unpredictable food supply.

As human societies progressed, fasting took on new roles and meanings. Many ancient cultures and religions incorporated fasting into their rituals and beliefs. For example, in ancient Greece, fasting was believed to enhance cognitive abilities and promote self-discipline. The Greek philosopher Plato once said, "I fast for greater physical and mental efficiency." He was not alone in this belief, as his student, Aristotle, also shared the view that fasting could improve mental clarity.

Religious fasting has also played a significant role in shaping the practice's history. In Christianity, fasting is a form of penance and spiritual cleansing. Jesus fasted for 40 days in the desert, a practice commemorated by Christians during Lent.

In Islam, the month-long fast of Ramadan is one of the Five Pillars of the faith. Observant Muslims abstain from food and drink from sunrise to sunset during this time to deepen their connection with God and cultivate empathy for the less fortunate. Similarly, fasting is practiced in Judaism during Yom Kippur and in Buddhism as a means to purify the mind and body.

In the 20th century, fasting gained new attention as a potential means to improve health and promote longevity. Dr. Yoshinori Ohsumi's groundbreaking research on autophagy, for which he received the Nobel Prize in Physiology or Medicine in 2016, demonstrated that fasting could activate cellular processes that help the body repair itself and remove damaged cells. This research reignited interest in the health benefits of fasting, leading to the development of various intermittent fasting methods.

Intermittent fasting, as we know it today, is a conscious and structured approach to incorporating fasting into one's lifestyle for health and wellness purposes. Unlike prolonged fasting, which can last for several days or weeks, intermittent fasting involves alternating periods of eating and fasting within a defined time frame. There are different types of intermittent fasting, such as the 16/8 method, where you fast for 16 hours and eat within an 8-hour window, or the 5:2 method, where you eat normally for five days and consume a reduced calorie intake on two non-consecutive days.

As we move through this book, we will delve into the science behind intermittent fasting, the various methods you can choose from, and the potential benefits and risks associated with this practice. By understanding the history and evolution of fasting, we can better appreciate the journey that has led to the intermittent fasting methods we have today. With this knowledge in hand, you will be well-equipped to make informed decisions about incorporating intermittent fasting into your own life.

Intermittent Fasting: An Overview

Intermittent fasting has become increasingly popular over the past decade as a powerful tool for managing weight, enhancing mental clarity, and improving overall health. Its simplicity and flexibility have made it appealing to a wide range of individuals looking for a sustainable and effective approach to healthy living. This chapter will provide an overview of intermittent fasting, including its various methods, benefits, and potential drawbacks, and how it can be incorporated into your daily routine.

The Basics of Intermittent Fasting

At its core, intermittent fasting involves alternating periods of eating and fasting. Unlike many other dietary approaches, intermittent fasting is not focused on the types of food you eat or specific macronutrient ratios, but rather on the timing of your meals. The rationale behind intermittent fasting is that by allowing your body to enter a fasting state regularly, you can tap into various physiological processes that promote overall health.

There are several methods of intermittent fasting, each with its own set of guidelines for eating and fasting periods. Some of the most popular methods include:

1. 16/8 Method: This involves fasting for 16 hours a day and eating during an 8-hour window. For example, you might eat between noon and 8 PM and fast from 8 PM to noon the following day.
2. 5:2 Method: This method involves eating normally for five days of the week and consuming only 500-600 calories on the remaining two non-consecutive days.
3. Eat-Stop-Eat: This approach involves fasting for 24 hours once or twice a week, with normal eating on the other days.
4. Alternate-Day Fasting: As the name suggests, this method involves fasting every other day, with normal eating on non-fasting days.

The Benefits of Intermittent Fasting

Intermittent fasting has been associated with numerous health benefits, supported by both scientific research and anecdotal evidence:

1. Weight Loss: By reducing the number of meals and total caloric intake, intermittent fasting can lead to weight loss. It also promotes fat burning by increasing the body's reliance on stored fat for energy during fasting periods.
2. Improved Insulin Sensitivity: Intermittent fasting may help improve insulin sensitivity and reduce the risk of type 2 diabetes by allowing the body to more effectively utilize glucose and regulate blood sugar levels.
3. Enhanced Mental Clarity: Many people report increased mental clarity and focus during fasting periods due to the effects of ketosis – a metabolic state where the body burns fat for fuel in the absence of glucose.
4. Cellular Repair and Longevity: Fasting may stimulate autophagy – the process by which cells remove and recycle damaged components, leading to improved cellular function and potentially increased longevity.
5. Reduced Inflammation: Intermittent fasting may help reduce inflammation and oxidative stress, both of which are associated with various chronic diseases.

Potential Drawbacks and Considerations

While intermittent fasting can offer significant health benefits, it's essential to be aware of potential drawbacks and to consider individual factors before adopting this lifestyle:

1. Hunger and Cravings: Intermittent fasting can be challenging, especially during the initial adjustment period when hunger and cravings might be more intense.
2. Social Considerations: Fasting periods may interfere with social events or family mealtimes, making it difficult to maintain this lifestyle.
3. Nutrient Intake: It's essential to ensure you're still getting adequate nutrients during your eating windows, especially if you're following more restrictive fasting methods.
4. Medical Conditions: People with certain medical conditions or those taking medications that require food intake should consult their healthcare provider before attempting intermittent fasting.

Incorporating Intermittent Fasting into Your Routine

If you're interested in trying intermittent fasting, it's important to choose a method that best suits your lifestyle, preferences, and goals. Begin by considering your daily schedule, social commitments, and personal preferences to determine which fasting method is most likely to be sustainable for you.

Here are some tips to help you incorporate intermittent fasting into your routine:

1. Start Slowly: If you're new to intermittent fasting, ease into it by gradually increasing your fasting periods. This can help you become more comfortable with the sensation of hunger and make the transition smoother.
2. Stay Hydrated: Drinking water, black coffee, or unsweetened tea during fasting periods can help keep you hydrated and may alleviate hunger pangs.
3. Prioritize Nutrition: Focus on consuming nutrient-dense foods during your eating windows to ensure you're getting all the essential vitamins, minerals, and macronutrients your body needs.
4. Listen to Your Body: If you're feeling unwell or notice any adverse effects from fasting, don't hesitate to modify your fasting schedule or consult a healthcare professional for guidance.
5. Combine with Physical Activity: Regular exercise can complement intermittent fasting by promoting weight loss, improving insulin sensitivity, and enhancing overall health.
6. Be Patient: It may take some time for your body to adjust to a new eating pattern. Give yourself time to adapt, and remember that consistency is key to reaping the benefits of intermittent fasting.

In conclusion, intermittent fasting is a flexible and potentially powerful approach to promoting overall health and wellness. By understanding the basics, benefits, and potential drawbacks, you can make an informed decision about whether this lifestyle is right for you. And by incorporating intermittent fasting into your routine thoughtfully, you can set yourself up for success on your journey to improved health.

Health Benefits and Science-backed Research

Intermittent fasting (IF) has gained significant traction in recent years as a popular approach to weight management, improved health, and overall well-being. Rooted in a combination of traditional wisdom and modern scientific research, IF offers numerous health benefits backed by a growing body of evidence. In this chapter, we will delve into the science behind intermittent fasting, its various health benefits, and the current state of research supporting its effectiveness.

1. Weight Loss and Improved Metabolism

One of the most well-known benefits of intermittent fasting is its potential to aid in weight loss. By restricting eating to specific periods or limiting calorie intake on certain days, IF helps create a calorie deficit that promotes weight loss. Studies have demonstrated that IF can lead to a reduction in body weight, body fat, and waist circumference (1). Furthermore, IF has been shown to increase metabolic rate, thereby boosting the body's ability to burn calories more efficiently (2).

2. Enhanced Insulin Sensitivity and Reduced Blood Sugar Levels

Intermittent fasting has been shown to improve insulin sensitivity and reduce blood sugar levels. This can be particularly beneficial for individuals with type 2 diabetes or those at risk for developing the condition. Studies have shown that IF can reduce insulin resistance and lower fasting glucose levels, ultimately improving glycemic control (3). By enhancing insulin sensitivity, IF may also help in the prevention of type 2 diabetes.

3. Improved Cardiovascular Health

Emerging research suggests that IF can have a positive impact on cardiovascular health. Studies have demonstrated that IF may lead to reductions in total cholesterol, triglycerides, and LDL cholesterol (the "bad" cholesterol) while increasing HDL cholesterol (the "good" cholesterol) (4). These changes can lower the risk of developing heart disease and stroke. Additionally, IF has been shown to reduce blood pressure and inflammation, further contributing to improved cardiovascular health (5).

4. Enhanced Brain Health and Cognitive Function

Intermittent fasting may also provide benefits for brain health and cognitive function. Research has shown that IF can increase the production of brain-derived neurotrophic factor (BDNF), a protein that plays a crucial role in the growth and maintenance of neurons (6). Higher BDNF levels are associated with improved memory, learning, and overall cognitive function. Furthermore, IF has been shown to reduce oxidative stress and inflammation in the brain, potentially protecting against neurodegenerative diseases such as Alzheimer's and Parkinson's (7).

5. Increased Cellular Repair and Autophagy

Autophagy is a cellular process that involves the removal of damaged proteins and organelles, as well as the recycling of cellular components. IF has been shown to stimulate autophagy, thereby promoting cellular repair and maintaining cellular health (8). Increased autophagy may help protect against various diseases, including cancer and neurodegenerative conditions, by eliminating damaged cells and reducing inflammation (9).

While the benefits of intermittent fasting are promising, it is essential to recognize that more research is needed to fully understand the long-term effects and optimal approaches to IF. Individuals should consult with their healthcare provider before embarking on an intermittent fasting journey to ensure it is appropriate for their unique health needs and goals.

As we have explored the various health benefits and science-backed research supporting intermittent fasting, it is important to acknowledge that IF is not a one-size-fits-all approach. People's experiences with intermittent fasting can vary, and it may not be suitable for everyone. There are different methods of IF, such as the 16/8 method, the 5:2 method, and alternate-day fasting, which cater to different lifestyles and preferences. It is crucial to find the approach that best fits an individual's needs, goals, and medical conditions.

Moreover, certain populations should exercise caution before adopting intermittent fasting, such as pregnant or breastfeeding women, individuals with a history of eating disorders, and those with specific medical conditions. It is always recommended to consult a healthcare professional before starting an IF regimen to ensure it is safe and appropriate for one's circumstances.

In summary, intermittent fasting offers a range of science-backed health benefits, including weight loss, improved metabolism, enhanced insulin sensitivity, better cardiovascular health, increased brain function, and increased cellular repair through autophagy. While more research is needed to determine the long-term effects and optimal methods of IF, the current body of evidence supports its potential as a valuable tool in promoting overall health and well-being.

References:
1. Varady, K. A. (2011). Intermittent versus daily calorie restriction: which diet regimen is more effective for weight loss? Obesity Reviews, 12(7), e593-e601.
2. Zauner, C., Schneeweiss, B., Kranz, A., Madl, C., Ratheiser, K., & Kramer, L. (2000). Resting energy expenditure in short-term starvation is increased as a result of an increase in serum norepinephrine. The American Journal of Clinical Nutrition71(6), 1511-1515.
3. Patterson, R. E., & Sears, D. D. (2017). Metabolic Effects of Intermittent Fasting. Annual Review of Nutrition, 37, 371-393.
4. Horne, B. D., Muhlestein, J. B., & Anderson, J. L. (2015). Health effects of intermittent fasting: hormesis or harm? A systematic review. The American Journal of Clinical Nutrition, 102(2), 464-470.

5. de Cabo, R., & Mattson, M. P. (2019). Effects of Intermittent Fasting on Health, Aging, and Disease. New England Journal of Medicine, 381(26), 2541-2551.

6. Mattson, M. P., & Arumugam, T. V. (2018). Hallmarks of Brain Aging: Adaptive and Pathological Modification by Metabolic States. Cell Metabolism, 27(6), 1176-1199.

7. Liguori, I., Russo, G., Curcio, F., Bulli, G., Aran, L., Della-Morte, D., & Abete, P. (2018). Oxidative stress, aging, and diseases. Clinical Interventions in Aging, 13, 757-772.

8. Rubinsztein, D. C., Mariño, G., & Kroemer, G. (2011). Autophagy and aging. Cell, 146(5), 682-695.

9. White, E., & DiPaola, R. S. (2009). The double-edged sword of autophagy modulation in cancer. Clinical Cancer Research, 15(17), 5308-5316.

Chapter 2: The Physiology of Fasting

The Metabolic Switch: Fasting vs. Feeding

In this chapter, we will delve deeper into the physiological aspects of fasting, particularly the metabolic switch that occurs between fasting and feeding states. Understanding the science behind fasting will help you appreciate its numerous health benefits and guide you on your intermittent fasting journey.

The human body is a remarkable machine that can seamlessly adapt to varying energy needs. When you consume food, your body breaks it down into its basic components, such as carbohydrates, proteins, and fats. These are then utilized to provide the energy necessary for maintaining essential bodily functions and fueling physical activities.

Feeding and fasting states induce different metabolic processes, with the body's energy source being the primary differentiator. Let's take a closer look at these two states and the metabolic switch that occurs between them.

Feeding State
When you eat, your body breaks down carbohydrates into glucose, which is the primary source of energy for your cells. Glucose enters the bloodstream, causing a rise in blood sugar levels. To manage this increase, the pancreas

releases insulin, a hormone that signals cells to absorb glucose from the bloodstream and convert it into glycogen or fat for storage.

In the feeding state, the body prioritizes using glucose for energy, and any excess is stored in the liver and muscles as glycogen or converted into fat in adipose tissue. This process is known as lipogenesis.

Fasting State

When you stop eating, your body needs to find alternative sources of energy as glucose levels in the bloodstream decrease. After about 12 hours of fasting, glycogen stores in the liver begin to deplete. To continue providing energy, the body initiates a process called glycogenolysis, where it breaks down glycogen into glucose.

As fasting continues, the body shifts to a state of ketosis, where it starts to burn fat for fuel instead of glucose. The liver converts fatty acids into ketone bodies, which can be used by most cells, including the brain, as an alternative energy source. This process is known as lipolysis.

The Metabolic Switch

The metabolic switch refers to the transition between the feeding state (relying primarily on glucose for energy) and the fasting state (using ketone bodies and fatty acids as primary energy sources). This switch is a natural process that has been critical to human survival during times of food scarcity.

Intermittent fasting promotes this metabolic switch by allowing your body to cycle between periods of feeding and fasting. By doing so, you're essentially training your body to become more efficient at burning fat for energy. This adaptation can have several health benefits, including weight loss, improved insulin sensitivity, and enhanced cellular repair processes.

In the next sections, we will explore the physiological changes that occur during fasting, including hormonal shifts, cellular repair mechanisms, and the impact of fasting on inflammation and immunity. These insights will help you appreciate the science behind intermittent fasting and how it can lead to improved health and wellness.

Hormones and Intermittent Fasting

Intermittent fasting (IF) has grown in popularity over the years as an effective approach to weight loss and overall health improvement. One of the reasons behind its success lies in its ability to positively influence hormone production and regulation in our bodies. Hormones play a crucial role in regulating various bodily functions such as metabolism, hunger, mood, and sleep. In this chapter, we will delve into the fascinating world of hormones and how intermittent fasting can help optimize their levels and improve our overall well-being.

1. Insulin

Insulin is a key hormone responsible for regulating blood sugar levels. It facilitates the uptake of glucose (sugar) into our cells, where it is either used for energy or stored as fat. When we eat, our insulin levels rise to manage the influx of glucose. However, frequent and excessive insulin spikes can lead to insulin resistance, where our cells become less responsive to the hormone. This condition often precedes type 2 diabetes and is associated with weight gain and obesity.

Intermittent fasting helps improve insulin sensitivity by allowing the body to take breaks from constant insulin production. During fasting periods, insulin levels drop, promoting fat burning and reducing the risk of developing insulin resistance. Many studies have shown that intermittent fasting can be an effective strategy to manage blood sugar levels and prevent type 2 diabetes.

2. Human Growth Hormone (HGH)

Human growth hormone (HGH) is primarily involved in growth, cell regeneration, and cell reproduction. It plays a vital role in maintaining muscle mass, bone density, and metabolism. HGH production typically declines as we age, contributing to muscle loss, fat gain, and a slower metabolism.

Intermittent fasting can stimulate the release of HGH, thereby enhancing muscle growth, promoting fat burning, and boosting metabolism. Fasting periods create a favorable environment for HGH production by reducing insulin levels and increasing levels of other hormones that promote HGH release, such as ghrelin.

3. Ghrelin

Ghrelin, often referred to as the "hunger hormone," is responsible for regulating appetite. It signals the brain to stimulate feelings of hunger when the body needs energy. Although it may seem counterintuitive, intermittent fasting can help control ghrelin levels and reduce hunger sensations over time.

During the initial stages of intermittent fasting, ghrelin levels may increase, causing hunger pangs. However, as the body adapts to the fasting routine, ghrelin levels stabilize, leading to reduced hunger sensations and improved appetite control. This makes it easier to adhere to intermittent fasting and maintain a healthy weight.

4. Leptin

Leptin, known as the "satiety hormone," is produced by fat cells and helps regulate energy balance by signaling the brain when we have had enough food. Leptin resistance, where the brain doesn't respond to leptin signals, can lead to overeating and weight gain.

Intermittent fasting has been shown to improve leptin sensitivity, helping the brain better recognize satiety signals and prevent overeating. By enhancing leptin sensitivity, intermittent fasting can contribute to long-term weight management and overall health.

5. Cortisol

Cortisol is a stress hormone that plays a role in various bodily functions, including blood sugar regulation and inflammation. While it is essential for survival, chronically elevated cortisol levels can lead to weight gain, insulin resistance, and other health issues.

Intermittent fasting may help regulate cortisol levels by promoting a more balanced and stable hormonal environment. Studies have shown that practicing intermittent fasting can lower cortisol levels, reducing stress and promoting overall well-being.

Hormones are essential messengers in our bodies, orchestrating various physiological processes that contribute to our health. Intermittent fasting has the potential to optimize hormone levels, offering numerous health benefits such as improved insulin sensitivity, increased HGH production, better appetite regulation, enhanced leptin sensitivity, and reduced cortisol levels.

By positively impacting these hormones, intermittent fasting can promote weight loss, improve metabolic health, and enhance overall well-being.

It is important to note that individual responses to intermittent fasting may vary, and it may not be suitable for everyone. Before embarking on an intermittent fasting journey, consult with a healthcare professional to determine if it is an appropriate strategy for your unique health goals and circumstances.

As we have explored in this chapter, hormones play a critical role in our health, and understanding their functions can empower us to make informed decisions about our well-being. Intermittent fasting is a promising approach that can help us harness the power of our hormones to achieve optimal health.

By adopting a balanced and sustainable fasting routine, we can potentially unlock numerous benefits and improve our quality of life.

Autophagy: Cellular Repair and Renewal

When it comes to intermittent fasting, one of the most fascinating and essential processes that takes place within our body is autophagy. This natural and highly efficient mechanism not only keeps our cells in optimal shape but also contributes to overall health and longevity. In this chapter, we will explore the intricacies of autophagy, how it links to intermittent fasting, and the role it plays in cellular repair and renewal.

The word "autophagy" originates from the Greek words "auto" (self) and "phagy" (to eat), and as the name suggests, it is a process where cells essentially "eat" themselves. However, this self-devouring should not be viewed negatively. Autophagy is a crucial cellular maintenance system that disposes of damaged, dysfunctional, or excess components. This cellular recycling system ultimately allows the cells to create new, healthy components and helps to maintain overall cellular health.

1. The Process of Autophagy

Autophagy can be broken down into three main steps: initiation, elongation, and degradation. During initiation, the cell identifies damaged or unnecessary components that need to be removed. Next, during elongation, a structure called the autophagosome forms around these components, encapsulating them in a double-layered membrane. Finally, the autophagosome fuses with a lysosome, an organelle filled with enzymes that break down and degrade the contents, effectively recycling the components back into the cell.

2. Autophagy and Intermittent Fasting

You may be wondering how autophagy relates to intermittent fasting. The answer lies in the fact that fasting stimulates the autophagy process. When you fast, your body experiences a decrease in nutrient availability and an increase in cellular stress. This triggers a series of molecular pathways that ultimately promote autophagy.

During intermittent fasting, your body undergoes periods of feast and famine. The famine phase, when you are not consuming any calories, is when autophagy ramps up. The process of intermittent fasting, therefore, serves as a natural and effective way to stimulate autophagy, which in turn enhances cellular repair and renewal.

3. **Benefits of Autophagy**

The role of autophagy in cellular repair and renewal is paramount, and the benefits of this process extend beyond just keeping our cells in good shape. Here are some of the key advantages associated with autophagy:

- Disease prevention: Autophagy helps prevent neurodegenerative diseases like Alzheimer's and Parkinson's by clearing out damaged proteins and organelles. It also plays a role in reducing inflammation and preventing diseases like cancer and cardiovascular disorders.
- Improved immune function: By clearing out pathogens and damaged cellular components, autophagy boosts our body's natural immune response.
- Enhanced longevity: Studies have shown that increased autophagy is linked to a longer, healthier life. By maintaining healthy cellular function, autophagy helps combat the aging process.
- Weight loss and metabolic health: Autophagy promotes the breakdown of stored fats and helps regulate glucose levels, ultimately leading to weight loss and improved metabolic health.

Autophagy is an essential cellular process that not only helps maintain cellular health but also plays a critical role in disease prevention, immune function, and longevity.

By engaging in intermittent fasting, we can harness the power of autophagy to promote cellular repair and renewal, ultimately contributing to a healthier, more vibrant life.

Chapter 3: Different Intermittent Fasting Methods

In this chapter, we will explore the various intermittent fasting methods that you can choose from to incorporate into your lifestyle. Each method has its own unique benefits and challenges, so it's essential to find the one that resonates with your goals and personal preferences. We will begin by delving into the 16/8 method, which is one of the most popular forms of intermittent fasting.

The 16/8 Method

The 16/8 method, also known as the Leangains protocol, is perhaps the most widely practiced and well-known intermittent fasting method. It involves fasting for 16 hours each day and restricting your eating window to 8 hours.

This method was popularized by Martin Berkhan, a Swedish nutritionist and personal trainer, who designed it as a simple yet effective way to lose weight, gain muscle, and improve overall health.

How does the 16/8 method work?
In the 16/8 method, you select an 8-hour eating window during which you consume all your daily calories. For example, if you choose to eat between noon and 8 PM, you would fast from 8 PM until noon the next day.

The beauty of the 16/8 method is its flexibility – you can adjust your eating window to suit your lifestyle and preferences.

Benefits of the 16/8 method:
1. Weight loss: With a restricted eating window, you're likely to consume fewer calories, which can lead to weight loss. Moreover, fasting for 16 hours allows your body to enter a fat-burning state, as it depletes glycogen stores and shifts to burning fat for fuel.
2. Improved insulin sensitivity: Intermittent fasting has been shown to improve insulin sensitivity, which helps your body use glucose more effectively. This may lower your risk of developing type 2 diabetes.
3. Enhanced brain health: Fasting can stimulate the production of brain-derived neurotrophic factor (BDNF), a protein that promotes the growth and maintenance of neurons. Higher BDNF levels are associated with better cognitive function and a reduced risk of neurodegenerative diseases.
4. Increased human growth hormone (HGH) levels: Fasting can boost HGH production, which plays a crucial role in muscle growth, fat loss, and cellular repair.
5. Autophagy: Intermittent fasting stimulates autophagy, a cellular process that breaks down and recycles damaged proteins and organelles. This may help protect against age-related diseases and improve overall cellular health.

Challenges and considerations:

1. Hunger: Adjusting to the 16/8 method may cause temporary hunger pangs, especially during the initial stages. However, this usually subsides as your body adapts to the new eating pattern.
2. Overeating: Some individuals may be tempted to overeat during their 8-hour eating window to compensate for the fasting period. To avoid this, focus on nutrient-dense, whole foods that keep you feeling full and satisfied.
3. Social events: The 16/8 method can sometimes interfere with social events that involve food. Be prepared to adjust your eating window or practice flexibility when it comes to occasional celebrations and gatherings.

In conclusion, the 16/8 method is an excellent option for those seeking a simple and flexible intermittent fasting approach.

It has been shown to promote weight loss, improve insulin sensitivity, and provide numerous other health benefits.

As with any lifestyle change, it's essential to listen to your body and consult with a healthcare professional before making any significant dietary modifications.

The 5:2 Diet

In this section, we'll explore the ins and outs of the 5:2 diet, its potential benefits, how to implement it, and the scientific research supporting its efficacy. So, grab a cup of tea, sit back, and let's dive into the world of the 5:2 diet.

What is the 5:2 Diet?

The 5:2 diet, also known as the Fast Diet, is an intermittent fasting method that involves eating normally for five days of the week and restricting caloric intake on two non-consecutive days.

On the fasting days, women typically consume around 500 calories, while men consume approximately 600 calories. This creates a calorie deficit that, over time, can lead to weight loss and other health benefits.

The 5:2 diet was popularized by Dr. Michael Mosley, a British physician and journalist, who documented his personal experience with the diet in a BBC documentary and subsequent book.

Benefits of the 5:2 Diet

1. Weight loss: The primary goal of the 5:2 diet for many is weight loss. By reducing calorie intake on fasting days, individuals create a calorie deficit that can lead to shedding unwanted pounds.
2. Improved insulin sensitivity: Intermittent fasting, including the 5:2 diet, has been shown to improve insulin sensitivity. This can help reduce the risk of

type 2 diabetes and support healthy blood sugar levels.

3. Enhanced brain health: Studies suggest that intermittent fasting may improve brain function and protect against age-related cognitive decline. This is thought to occur because fasting increases the production of brain-derived neurotrophic factor (BDNF), a protein that supports brain health.

4. Increased longevity: Research indicates that intermittent fasting may help to extend lifespan by promoting cellular repair processes and reducing inflammation.

5. Simplified meal planning: Many people find the 5:2 diet easier to follow than traditional calorie-restricted diets because it only requires strict adherence on two days per week.

Implementing the 5:2 Diet

1. Choose your fasting days: Select two non-consecutive days each week to be your fasting days. It's important to separate these days by at least one non-fasting day to allow your body time to recover.

2. Plan your meals: On fasting days, focus on consuming nutrient-dense, low-calorie foods, such as lean proteins, vegetables, and whole grains. Stay well-hydrated by drinking plenty of water, herbal teas, and black coffee.

3. Monitor your hunger levels: Hunger may be more noticeable on fasting days, but it's important to remember that it's temporary. Over time, your body will adjust to the new eating pattern.

4. Stay active: Incorporate light to moderate exercise into your routine on fasting days, but be cautious not to overdo it. Exercise can help you feel more energized and focused.
5. Listen to your body: The 5:2 diet is not suitable for everyone. If you experience extreme fatigue, dizziness, or other concerning symptoms, it's essential to consult your healthcare professional.

Scientific Evidence

Numerous studies have investigated the potential benefits of intermittent fasting and the 5:2 diet. While more research is needed, current findings show promising results in terms of weight loss, improved insulin sensitivity, and other health markers.

As always, it's important to consult with a healthcare professional before starting any new diet or lifestyle change.

In Conclusion

The 5:2 diet offers a flexible and sustainable approach to intermittent fasting that can be easily incorporated into most people's lifestyles.

By dedicating two non-consecutive days each week to restricted caloric intake, individuals can potentially reap the benefits of weight loss, improved insulin sensitivity, enhanced brain health, and increased longevity.

As with any dietary change, it's crucial to monitor your body's response and seek professional guidance when needed. If the 5:2 diet aligns with your personal goals and lifestyle, it can be an effective and enjoyable way to improve your overall health and well-being.

Remember, the key to successful long-term health outcomes is finding an approach that works for you and is sustainable in the long run.

While the 5:2 diet has garnered significant attention and produced promising results for many, it's important to consider your personal needs, preferences, and medical history when selecting the best dietary approach for you.

The Eat-Stop Method

What is the Eat-Stop Method?
The Eat-Stop Method is a form of intermittent fasting that involves alternating periods of eating with periods of fasting. Unlike other intermittent fasting protocols, such as the 16:8 or 5:2 methods, the Eat-Stop Method focuses on a more flexible approach, allowing individuals to adapt the fasting periods to their lifestyle and needs.

This method requires you to eat normally during your chosen eating window, followed by a fasting window that typically ranges from 12 to 24 hours, depending on your personal preferences and goals.

Benefits of the Eat-Stop Method

1. Weight Loss: One of the most compelling benefits of the Eat-Stop Method is weight loss. By restricting the eating window, you naturally reduce your overall caloric intake, which can lead to weight loss over time. Additionally, the fasting periods help improve insulin sensitivity, which allows the body to more effectively burn stored fat.

2. Improved Digestion: Fasting gives your digestive system a break, allowing it to recover and perform more efficiently when you resume eating. This can lead to improved digestion, reduced bloating, and a general feeling of lightness and well-being.

3. Enhanced Mental Clarity: Many individuals who practice the Eat-Stop Method report increased mental clarity and focus during the fasting periods. This is likely due to the increased production of ketones, which provide an alternative fuel source for the brain.

4. Cellular Repair and Autophagy: Fasting has been shown to trigger a process called autophagy, where the body breaks down and recycles damaged cells, proteins, and other cellular components. This process is essential for maintaining optimal cellular health and may help protect against various age-related diseases.

5. Increased Longevity: Research suggests that intermittent fasting, including the Eat-Stop Method, may contribute to increased longevity by promoting cellular repair, reducing inflammation, and improving metabolic health.

Implementing the Eat-Stop Method

Before embarking on the Eat-Stop Method, it's essential to consult with a healthcare professional to ensure it's appropriate for your individual needs and health status. Once you've gotten the green light, follow these steps to incorporate the Eat-Stop Method into your routine:

1. Choose your eating and fasting windows: Determine the length of your eating and fasting windows based on your lifestyle, goals, and personal preferences. Start with shorter fasting periods and gradually increase the duration as you become more comfortable with the process.
2. Plan your meals: During your eating window, aim for balanced and nutrient-dense meals that provide adequate protein, healthy fats, and complex carbohydrates. This will help maintain energy levels, support muscle growth and repair, and keep you satiated during the fasting periods.
3. Stay hydrated: Drinking water, herbal tea, and black coffee (without sugar or cream) is allowed during fasting periods and can help curb hunger, improve digestion, and maintain hydration.
4. Listen to your body: The Eat-Stop Method should be flexible and adaptable to your individual needs. If you find the fasting periods too challenging, consider adjusting the duration or frequency to better suit your lifestyle and health goals.
5. Combine with physical activity: Engaging in regular physical activity can help enhance the benefits of

the Eat-Stop Method, including weight loss and improved overall health.

The Eat-Stop Method offers a flexible and sustainable approach to intermittent fasting that can be tailored to individual needs and preferences. By incorporating this method into your lifestyle, you may experience a range of benefits, including weight loss, improved digestion, enhanced mental clarity, cellular repair, and increased longevity.

It's important to remember that the Eat-Stop Method may not be suitable for everyone, and it's always recommended to consult with a healthcare professional before making any significant changes to your diet or lifestyle.

As with any health and wellness journey, it's crucial to be patient, listen to your body, and find a balance that works best for you. With time, dedication, and proper planning, the Eat-Stop Method can become a valuable tool in achieving and maintaining optimal health and well-being.

Alternate-Day Fasting

Alternate-day fasting (ADF) is a popular form of intermittent fasting that has garnered significant attention in recent years. This type of fasting involves alternating between days of unrestricted eating and days of consuming a very low-calorie intake or fasting entirely.

As with other intermittent fasting methods, ADF aims to promote health benefits such as weight loss, improved metabolic health, and increased longevity. In this chapter, we will delve into the world of alternate-day fasting, discussing its mechanics, benefits, potential drawbacks, and practical tips to help you implement this fasting regimen effectively.

The Mechanics of Alternate-Day Fasting

The premise of ADF is quite simple: on fasting days, you consume little to no calories, while on non-fasting days, you eat without any restrictions. A common approach to ADF is to limit calorie intake to about 500 calories on fasting days, although some variations involve complete fasting.

The non-fasting days do not require any specific caloric or macronutrient restrictions, but it's essential to maintain a balanced and nutritious diet to maximize the health benefits of ADF. Consuming whole, unprocessed foods, such as vegetables, fruits, lean proteins, and healthy fats, should be prioritized on non-fasting days.

Benefits of Alternate-Day Fasting

1. Weight Loss: One of the primary motivations for adopting ADF is weight loss. By reducing calorie intake on fasting days, individuals can achieve a caloric deficit, leading to weight loss. Studies have shown that ADF can be an effective strategy for weight loss, with participants losing up to 7% of their body weight over a 12-week period.

2. Improved Metabolic Health: ADF has been shown to improve various markers of metabolic health, such as insulin sensitivity, blood sugar levels, and lipid profiles. These improvements can help reduce the risk of developing chronic conditions such as type 2 diabetes and cardiovascular disease.

3. Increased Longevity: Animal studies have suggested that ADF may increase lifespan by inducing cellular repair processes and reducing inflammation. Although more research is needed in humans, preliminary findings indicate that ADF may have potential longevity benefits.

Potential Drawbacks and Precautions

While ADF can offer numerous health benefits, it may not be suitable for everyone. Some potential drawbacks and precautions to consider include:

1. Adherence: The restrictive nature of ADF may be challenging for some individuals to maintain long-term. It's important to consider your lifestyle and personal preferences when choosing a fasting regimen to ensure long-term adherence and success.

2. Nutrient Deficiency: Limiting calorie intake on fasting days may increase the risk of nutrient deficiencies, especially if the non-fasting days are not nutritionally balanced. It's essential to prioritize nutrient-dense foods on non-fasting days to ensure adequate nutrient intake.

3. Disordered Eating Patterns: ADF may not be suitable for individuals with a history of disordered

eating, as the fasting days could trigger unhealthy eating behaviors or exacerbate existing issues.

4. Medical Conditions: Individuals with certain medical conditions or those taking medications should consult a healthcare professional before starting ADF, as it may not be suitable or may require adjustments to medication regimens.

Practical Tips for Implementing Alternate-Day Fasting

1. Start Slowly: If you're new to fasting, consider starting with a less restrictive form of intermittent fasting, such as the 16:8 method, and gradually progress to ADF to help your body adjust to the changes.

2. Stay Hydrated: On fasting days, it's crucial to stay well-hydrated. Drink plenty of water, and consider consuming calorie-free beverages like black coffee or herbal tea to help curb hunger.

3. Prioritize Sleep: Ensuring adequate sleep is essential during ADF, as sleep deprivation can exacerbate feelings of hunger and negatively impact your overall health. Aim for 7-9 hours of quality sleep each night to support your fasting regimen.

4. Plan Your Meals: On non-fasting days, focus on consuming nutrient-dense foods that provide a balance of protein, healthy fats, and complex carbohydrates. This will help ensure you receive adequate nutrition and maintain energy levels throughout your fasting regimen.

5. Listen to Your Body: If you experience extreme fatigue, dizziness, or other concerning symptoms during ADF, consult with a healthcare professional. It's essential to prioritize your well-being and adjust your fasting routine as needed.

6. Exercise Wisely: While it's generally safe to continue your regular exercise routine during ADF, consider adjusting the intensity or timing of your workouts to coincide with your non-fasting days, when you'll have more energy and fuel for your activities.

7. Be Mindful of Your Eating Habits: On non-fasting days, it's crucial to avoid overeating or indulging in unhealthy foods as a reward for fasting. Instead, practice mindful eating and focus on nourishing your body with wholesome, nutritious meals.

8. Track Your Progress: Keep a journal or use a smartphone app to track your fasting days, weight changes, and any improvements in your health markers. This can help you stay motivated and make adjustments to your fasting regimen if needed.

In conclusion, alternate-day fasting is a versatile and potentially effective form of intermittent fasting that can offer numerous health benefits, including weight loss and improved metabolic health.

However, it's essential to consider the potential drawbacks and precautions before embarking on this fasting journey.

By following the practical tips provided in this chapter, you can successfully implement ADF into your lifestyle and reap the rewards of this powerful health practice.

The Warrior Diet

The Warrior Diet is a unique form of intermittent fasting that has gained popularity over the years. This diet, which was popularized by Ori Hofmekler in his book of the same name, is based on the premise that our ancient ancestors, the warriors and hunters, used to eat only one substantial meal a day, typically in the evening.

In this section, we'll dive into the Warrior Diet, its principles, potential benefits, and practical tips for incorporating it into your life.

Origins and Principles

The Warrior Diet draws inspiration from ancient warrior societies, such as the Spartans and Roman soldiers, who are believed to have spent their days training and engaging in physical activities while consuming minimal amounts of food. The diet is based on the idea that our bodies are naturally adapted to function optimally on this kind of eating pattern.

The Warrior Diet is characterized by a 20-hour fasting window and a 4-hour eating window. During the fasting period, followers consume minimal amounts of food, focusing primarily on small portions of raw fruits, vegetables, and some protein sources.

In the eating window, dieters are encouraged to eat a large, nutrient-dense meal, often consisting of high-quality proteins, healthy fats, and complex carbohydrates.

Potential Benefits

1. Weight loss: The Warrior Diet may contribute to weight loss by creating a calorie deficit. The restricted eating window makes it more challenging to consume excess calories, which can lead to weight loss over time.
2. Improved insulin sensitivity: Intermittent fasting, including the Warrior Diet, has been shown to help regulate blood sugar levels and improve insulin sensitivity. This can be particularly beneficial for individuals with insulin resistance or type 2 diabetes.
3. Enhanced mental clarity: Fasting can help improve mental clarity and focus by increasing the production of brain-derived neurotrophic factor (BDNF). BDNF is a protein that supports the growth and survival of brain cells, leading to better cognitive function.
4. Autophagy: During extended fasting periods, the body undergoes a process called autophagy, where it cleanses itself of damaged cells and cellular waste. This process is believed to contribute to better overall health and longevity.

5. Potential hormonal benefits: The Warrior Diet may help regulate hormones such as growth hormone and cortisol, contributing to increased muscle mass, improved sleep quality, and reduced stress levels.

Practical Tips for Success

1. Stay hydrated: During the fasting window, make sure to drink plenty of water, herbal teas, or black coffee (without sugar or cream). Proper hydration is essential for overall health and can help curb hunger.
2. Prioritize nutrient-dense foods: When breaking your fast, choose high-quality, nutrient-dense foods to maximize the benefits of your eating window. Focus on lean proteins, healthy fats, and complex carbohydrates.
3. Gradually ease into the diet: If you're new to intermittent fasting, it can be helpful to gradually increase your fasting window rather than jumping straight into a 20-hour fast. This allows your body to adjust to the new eating pattern.
4. Listen to your body: While the Warrior Diet has many potential benefits, it's essential to listen to your body and adjust as needed. If you experience extreme fatigue, dizziness, or other negative symptoms, consult a healthcare professional and consider modifying the fasting window or approach.
5. Combine with regular exercise: For optimal results, incorporate regular physical activity into your

routine. This will not only support weight loss efforts but also improve overall health and well-being.

The Warrior Diet is an intriguing form of intermittent fasting that draws upon the eating habits of ancient warrior societies.

While this approach may not be suitable for everyone, it offers potential benefits such as weight loss, improved insulin sensitivity, enhanced mental clarity, and increased autophagy.

Finding Your Ideal Fasting Method

Intermittent fasting has gained immense popularity in recent years as a weight loss and health improvement strategy. With various methods and approaches to choose from, it can be a daunting task to find the one that works best for you. Let's guide you through the process of discovering your ideal fasting method, ensuring that it aligns with your lifestyle, goals, and personal preferences.

1. Understanding the Different Fasting Methods

Before you can select the perfect fasting method, it's essential to familiarize yourself with the most popular approaches.

Just to recap, here are some of the most common intermittent fasting methods:

- The 16/8 Method: This approach involves fasting for 16 hours each day and eating within an 8-hour window. For example, if you start eating at 12 PM, you would stop eating at 8 PM and then fast until 12 PM the next day.
- The 5:2 Method: With this method, you eat normally for five days a week and consume only 500-600 calories on the remaining two non-consecutive days.
- The Eat-Stop-Eat Method: This involves fasting for a full 24 hours once or twice a week.
- The Alternate-Day Fasting Method: As the name suggests, you alternate between fasting days (consuming only 500-600 calories) and regular eating days.
- The Warrior Diet: This method involves consuming minimal calories during the day and having a large meal at night, typically within a 4-hour eating window.

2. Assess Your Lifestyle and Goals

To find the best fasting method for you, consider your daily routine, work schedule, family commitments, and social life. Ask yourself the following questions:

- Can I easily incorporate fasting into my daily routine?
- Will my work or family life be affected by my fasting schedule?
- Can I maintain my social life while fasting?

Once you have a clear understanding of your lifestyle and commitments, consider your goals for intermittent fasting:

- Are you looking to lose weight, improve your overall health, or both?
- Are you aiming for short-term results or long-term health benefits?

3. Experiment with Different Methods

Everyone's body and experience with fasting are unique. It's essential to try different methods and observe how your body responds. Start with the method that seems most compatible with your lifestyle and goals, and give it a trial period of at least two weeks.

Keep a journal during this time to track your energy levels, mood, hunger, and any changes in weight or body composition. If you're not satisfied with the results or find it difficult to adhere to the fasting schedule, try another method until you find the one that works best for you.

4. Personalize Your Fasting Method

Once you've found the fasting method that suits your needs, you can make adjustments to further tailor it to your preferences. For example, if you're following the 16/8 method but prefer eating breakfast, you can shift your eating window to accommodate that.

5. Seek Professional Guidance

If you're unsure about which fasting method is best for you or have pre-existing health conditions, consult with a healthcare professional or registered dietitian. They can provide personalized recommendations based on your health history, current health status, and goals.

In conclusion, finding your ideal fasting method is a personal journey that requires experimentation and self-awareness.

By understanding the different fasting methods, assessing your lifestyle and goals, and being open to adjustments, you'll be well on your way to discovering the perfect intermittent fasting approach for you.

Remember, patience and consistency are key to reaping the benefits of this powerful health strategy.

Chapter 4: Combining Intermittent Fasting with Nutrition

Macronutrients and Micronutrients

Intermittent fasting (IF) has gained immense popularity in recent years due to its potential health benefits and weight loss results. However, to maximize the effectiveness of IF and ensure your body stays nourished and healthy, it's essential to combine it with proper nutrition.

In this chapter, we'll explore the importance of macronutrients and micronutrients in your diet and how to incorporate them effectively while practicing intermittent fasting.

Macronutrients are the main components of our diet, providing energy and essential nutrients for growth, development, and overall health. They include carbohydrates, proteins, and fats. Micronutrients, on the other hand, are vitamins and minerals required in smaller amounts, but are vital for maintaining proper bodily functions and preventing deficiencies.

Carbohydrates are the body's primary source of energy. They can be found in various food sources, such as grains, fruits, vegetables, and legumes. When practicing IF, it's crucial to consume complex carbohydrates, which are slowly digested, providing a steady energy supply throughout the fasting period. Examples of complex carbohydrates include whole grains, such as brown rice, quinoa, and whole-wheat products, as well as starchy vegetables like sweet potatoes and legumes.

Proteins are essential for building and repairing tissues, creating enzymes, and supporting immune function. High-quality protein sources include lean meats, poultry, fish, eggs, dairy products, legumes, nuts, and seeds. When following an IF regimen, it's important to consume adequate protein to maintain muscle mass and support your body's essential functions.

Fats are a vital component of a healthy diet, providing energy, supporting cell growth, and assisting in the absorption of essential fat-soluble vitamins.

There are three types of fats: saturated, unsaturated, and trans fats. Focus on consuming unsaturated fats, found in foods like avocados, nuts, seeds, and olive oil, while minimizing saturated and trans fats, which can contribute to heart disease and other health problems.

Now let's discuss micronutrients, which, despite being needed in smaller quantities, play a critical role in our health.
Micronutrients include essential vitamins and minerals, such as vitamins A, C, D, E, and K, as well as minerals like calcium, magnesium, potassium, and iron.

Vitamins play various roles in the body, such as supporting immune function, maintaining healthy skin and eyes, and aiding in blood clotting. Minerals are involved in processes like bone and teeth formation, muscle function, and maintaining fluid balance.

To ensure you're getting adequate micronutrients while practicing intermittent fasting, aim to consume a variety of nutrient-dense foods, such as colorful fruits and vegetables, whole grains, lean proteins, and healthy fats. Additionally, consider taking a daily multivitamin to fill in any nutritional gaps.

Combining intermittent fasting with a well-balanced, nutrient-dense diet is crucial for optimizing health, performance, and weight management. By paying close attention to your macronutrient and micronutrient intake, you can help support your body's essential functions and make the most of your IF journey.

Food Choices for Optimal Results

Now let's explore specific dietary strategies to optimize your intermittent fasting experience and the best food choices to optimize your results and support your overall health.

1. Prioritize Whole Foods

Aim to consume a diet primarily made up of whole foods. These are unprocessed or minimally processed items, such as fruits, vegetables, whole grains, legumes, nuts, seeds, and lean proteins.

Whole foods are nutrient-dense, providing the essential vitamins, minerals, and antioxidants your body needs to thrive. They also typically contain higher levels of dietary fiber, which aids in digestion, blood sugar regulation, and satiety.

2. Opt for High-Quality Protein Sources

Protein is a crucial macronutrient that supports muscle repair and growth, immune function, and hormone production. When choosing protein sources, consider options that are nutrient-rich and minimally processed. Examples include:

- Lean meats (e.g., chicken, turkey, or grass-fed beef)
- Fish (especially fatty fish like salmon, mackerel, and sardines, which are high in omega-3 fatty acids)
- Eggs
- Plant-based options like legumes, quinoa, tofu, tempeh, and edamame

3. Emphasize Healthy Fats

Contrary to popular belief, not all fats are bad for you. In fact, healthy fats play essential roles in hormone production, brain function, and nutrient absorption. Monounsaturated and polyunsaturated fats can also help lower inflammation and support heart health. Include the following healthy fats in your diet:

- Avocados
- Nuts (e.g., almonds, walnuts, and cashews)
- Seeds (e.g., chia, flax, and hemp)

- Olive oil and other cold-pressed oils
- Fatty fish (as mentioned earlier)

4. Choose Complex Carbohydrates

Carbohydrates are the body's primary source of energy, but not all carbs are created equal. Complex carbohydrates, like those found in whole grains, legumes, and starchy vegetables, are preferable to simple carbs like those in refined grains and sugar-laden products.

Complex carbs are digested more slowly, providing a steady source of energy and helping to stabilize blood sugar levels. Some great complex carbohydrate sources include:

- Whole grains (e.g., brown rice, quinoa, oats, and whole wheat)
- Legumes (e.g., beans, lentils, and chickpeas)
- Starchy vegetables (e.g., sweet potatoes, squash, and beets)

5. Hydration is Key

While intermittent fasting, it's crucial to stay adequately hydrated. Water plays a vital role in supporting digestion, metabolism, and nutrient absorption. Aim to drink at least eight 8-ounce glasses of water per day, or more if you're physically active or live in a hot climate.

6. Mind Your Micronutrients

Eating a varied and colorful diet will help ensure you consume a wide range of micronutrients (vitamins and minerals) that support optimal health. Fruits and vegetables are excellent sources of vitamins, minerals, and antioxidants. To maximize the benefits, aim to eat a rainbow of colors each day – think dark leafy greens, vibrant berries, and colorful bell peppers.

7. Limit Processed Foods and Added Sugars

While it's essential to focus on nutrient-dense foods, it's equally important to limit your intake of processed items and added sugars. Processed foods are often high in unhealthy fats, added sugars, and sodium, which can contribute to inflammation, weight gain, and chronic health issues. Limit your consumption of processed snacks, sugary beverages, and fast food, opting for whole food alternatives whenever possible.

8. Mindful Eating and Portion Control

Even with the best food choices, it's essential to practice mindful eating and be aware of portion sizes. Overeating, even healthy foods, can hinder your progress with intermittent fasting. Listen to your body's hunger and satiety cues, and try to eat slowly, savoring each bite. This can help prevent overeating and encourage a more enjoyable eating experience.

9. Customize Your Diet to Your Needs

While the guidelines provided in this chapter serve as a solid foundation, it's important to recognize that everyone's nutritional needs and preferences vary. Factors such as age, gender, activity level, and personal health conditions can influence your dietary requirements. Don't be afraid to tailor your food choices to your unique needs and preferences. You may also benefit from consulting a registered dietitian or nutritionist to help create a personalized meal plan that supports your intermittent fasting goals and overall health.

10. Flexibility and Balance

Finally, remember that maintaining a healthy diet doesn't require perfection. It's essential to allow yourself some flexibility and enjoy your favorite treats in moderation. Striving for balance and consistency in your food choices will promote long-term success with intermittent fasting and support a healthy, sustainable lifestyle.

In conclusion, the food choices you make during your eating window can significantly impact the success of your intermittent fasting journey.

By prioritizing whole foods, high-quality protein sources, healthy fats, complex carbohydrates, and a diverse array of micronutrients, you'll be providing your body with the essential nutrients it needs to function optimally.

In turn, this can amplify the benefits of intermittent fasting, such as improved weight management, increased energy levels, better cognitive function, and enhanced overall health.

By following these guidelines and making mindful, nutritious food choices during your eating window, you can maximize the benefits of intermittent fasting and improve your overall health and well-being.

Remember that everyone's journey is unique, and it's essential to be patient and compassionate with yourself as you navigate the world of intermittent fasting.

With time, consistency, and a focus on whole, nutrient-dense foods, you'll be well on your way to achieving your health and wellness goals.

Hydration and Electrolytes during Fasting

To reap the benefits of intermittent fasting while staying healthy and feeling great, it's essential to pay attention to hydration and electrolyte balance during the fasting period.

Let's dive (pun intended!) into the importance of hydration and electrolytes, discussing how they can impact your fasting experience and provide you with guidance on maintaining optimal levels.

The Importance of Hydration

Water is crucial for the proper functioning of the body. It aids in digestion, regulates body temperature, lubricates joints, transports nutrients, and removes waste products. Dehydration can result in a range of unpleasant symptoms like fatigue, dizziness, headache, and muscle cramps.

During fasting, it's crucial to stay properly hydrated since you may not be consuming water-rich foods or beverages.

Fasting can also cause a diuretic effect as the body starts to break down stored glycogen for energy, which leads to the loss of water weight.

This process can further increase the risk of dehydration if you're not conscious of your water intake. Aim for at least 8-10 glasses of water per day, but remember that individual needs may vary depending on factors like age, weight, physical activity, and climate.

Electrolytes: The Unsung Heroes
Electrolytes are minerals that dissolve in water and carry an electric charge, enabling them to regulate various functions within the body. The primary electrolytes are sodium, potassium, magnesium, calcium, and chloride. These essential minerals play a vital role in muscle contractions, nerve impulses, pH balance, and fluid regulation.

During fasting, electrolyte imbalances may occur as the body shifts to using stored fat for energy and starts shedding water weight. Symptoms of an electrolyte imbalance can include muscle cramps, irregular heartbeat, weakness, and even mental confusion.

To maintain optimal electrolyte levels, it's essential to be mindful of your intake, especially when fasting for extended periods.

Strategies for Maintaining Hydration and Electrolyte Balance

1. Drink water consistently: Make a habit of sipping water throughout the day, even if you're not thirsty. Set reminders or carry a water bottle with you as a visual cue to stay hydrated. Avoid excessive caffeine and alcohol consumption, as these can have a diuretic effect.
2. Add a pinch of salt: Adding a small amount of high-quality sea salt or Himalayan pink salt to your water can help replenish sodium levels. This can be particularly helpful during longer fasting periods or for those who exercise regularly.
3. Consume electrolyte-rich foods: During your eating window, consume foods rich in electrolytes, such as dark leafy greens, avocados, nuts, seeds, and yogurt. These foods will help replenish lost minerals and support overall health.
4. Use electrolyte supplements: In some cases, using an electrolyte supplement can be beneficial, especially for those who engage in intense physical activity or fast for extended periods. Look for supplements without added sugars or artificial ingredients.
5. Listen to your body: Pay attention to how you feel during your fast. If you experience symptoms of dehydration or electrolyte imbalances, adjust your hydration and electrolyte intake accordingly.

Staying hydrated and maintaining proper electrolyte balance are essential for a successful and healthy fasting experience.

By incorporating the strategies discussed in this chapter, you can support your body's functions, minimize unpleasant symptoms, and enhance the benefits of your intermittent fasting journey.

Chapter 5: Exercise and Intermittent Fasting

Benefits of Combining Exercise and Fasting

The science behind fasting and exercise is fascinating. When we fast, our bodies enter a state of energy conservation, tapping into stored fat for fuel. By exercising during this period, we can optimize fat burning, as well as other health benefits.

Here are some of the key advantages of combining exercise with intermittent fasting:

1. Enhanced Fat Loss: Both fasting and exercise stimulate lipolysis, the process of breaking down fats into smaller molecules that can be used for energy. When combined, these two factors can lead to a more efficient fat-burning process, helping you shed unwanted pounds.

2. Improved Insulin Sensitivity: Fasting and exercise have been shown to improve insulin sensitivity, which can be particularly helpful for those with insulin resistance or type 2 diabetes. By enhancing the body's ability to respond to insulin, you may be able to better control blood sugar levels and reduce the risk of diabetes-related complications.

3. Increased Human Growth Hormone (HGH) Production: Fasting and high-intensity exercise

both stimulate the release of HGH, a hormone that promotes muscle growth, fat loss, and tissue repair. By combining the two, you can potentially boost your HGH levels, leading to improved muscle tone and overall body composition.

4. Autophagy Activation: Autophagy is a cellular process that helps remove damaged or dysfunctional components within cells, promoting overall cellular health. Fasting has been shown to activate autophagy, and adding exercise to the mix may enhance this effect, contributing to a healthier, more resilient body.

5. Cardiovascular Health: Exercise is well-known for its heart-healthy benefits, and fasting may amplify these effects. Research suggests that IF can help reduce blood pressure, lower cholesterol levels, and improve overall cardiovascular health, making it a powerful combination for heart health.

6. Enhanced Cognitive Function: Both fasting and exercise have been linked to improvements in cognitive function, such as memory and learning. Combining the two might lead to even greater brain benefits, keeping your mind sharp and focused.

7. Boosted Immune System: Fasting and exercise can help strengthen the immune system by reducing inflammation and promoting the production of white blood cells. This powerful duo may help you ward off illness and recover more quickly from infections.

While the benefits of combining exercise and intermittent fasting are compelling, it's important to approach this combination with caution, especially if you're new to fasting or have pre-existing medical conditions. In the next section, we'll discuss how to safely integrate exercise into your fasting routine and provide tips for maximizing your results.

Best Exercise Regimes for Fasters

Let's explore the best exercise regimes for those practicing intermittent fasting, providing you with the tools and knowledge to get the most out of your fasted workouts.

Before diving into specific exercise regimes, let's take a moment to understand the benefits of exercising during your fasting window:

1. Enhanced Fat Loss: Exercising in a fasted state can increase fat oxidation, helping your body tap into stored fat for energy.
2. Improved Insulin Sensitivity: Fasted exercise can lead to better insulin sensitivity, allowing your body to process carbs more effectively and reducing the risk of diabetes.
3. Autophagy: Fasting and exercise can both trigger autophagy, the process by which your body clears out damaged cells and recycles cellular components.

Now that we've established the benefits, let's explore the best exercise regimes for fasters.

1. Low-Intensity Steady State Cardio (LISS)

Low-intensity steady state cardio, such as walking, cycling, or swimming, is an excellent choice for fasters. This type of exercise is gentle on your body and can be performed for extended periods without causing excessive stress. Moreover, LISS can help you burn fat while preserving muscle mass, a major concern for those on a weight loss journey.

Try incorporating 30-60 minutes of LISS into your fasting window at least three times a week. To keep things interesting, switch up your activities and explore different locations, like a nature trail or a scenic bike path.

2. High-Intensity Interval Training (HIIT)

High-intensity interval training consists of short, intense bursts of activity followed by periods of rest or low-intensity exercise. HIIT is a time-efficient way to improve cardiovascular fitness, increase fat loss, and maintain muscle mass. While it may seem counterintuitive to perform high-intensity exercises while fasting, many people find that they can handle HIIT workouts just fine in a fasted state.

Beginners can start with a 10-20 minute HIIT session two to three times a week, gradually increasing the intensity and duration as they become more comfortable.

An example of a HIIT workout could be alternating 30 seconds of sprinting with 90 seconds of walking, repeated for a total of 10-15 minutes.

3. Resistance Training

Resistance training, such as weightlifting or bodyweight exercises, is crucial for maintaining and building muscle mass, particularly while fasting. Strength training can also improve bone density and support a healthy metabolism.

Aim to perform resistance training two to three times a week, targeting all major muscle groups. You can either train in a fasted state or schedule your workouts closer to your eating window, depending on your personal preference and energy levels.

4. Restorative Practices

Don't forget to include restorative practices like yoga, Pilates, or stretching in your exercise regime. These activities can help improve flexibility, prevent injuries, and promote relaxation. Try incorporating one or two restorative sessions per week to support your overall well-being.

The key to finding the best exercise regime for you is to listen to your body and make adjustments as needed. While fasting can provide a unique opportunity to optimize your workouts for fat loss and health benefits, it's essential to prioritize self-care and recovery.

By combining intermittent fasting with a balanced exercise routine, you'll be well on your way to achieving your health and fitness goals.

Timing Your Workouts

When it comes to intermittent fasting and exercise, timing plays a crucial role in maximizing the benefits of both practices. Finding the perfect balance between your fasting window and your workouts can be a game-changer for your fitness journey.

The Importance of Timing

Timing your workouts during intermittent fasting can impact several factors, such as:

1. Energy levels: Many people find that their energy levels vary throughout their fasting window. By scheduling your workouts during the periods when you feel most energized, you can optimize your performance and prevent burnout.
2. Fat burning: Exercising during your fasting window may increase the rate at which your body burns fat for fuel, leading to more significant fat loss results.
3. Recovery: Properly timing your workouts can help you optimize post-workout recovery and ensure that you're adequately fueling your body to repair and rebuild muscle tissue.

Now that we understand the importance of workout timing, let's dive into some practical tips to help you optimize your exercise schedule.

1. Experiment with Different Timing

There is no one-size-fits-all solution when it comes to timing your workouts during intermittent fasting. Everyone's body is different, and what works for one person may not be ideal for another. To find the best time for your workouts, start by experimenting with different timings:

- Morning workouts: Some people prefer to exercise first thing in the morning, as they feel energized and focused. This can be particularly beneficial if you're practicing a 16:8 fasting protocol and finish eating around 8 p.m., as you'll be in a fasted state.
- Midday workouts: If you're following a longer fasting window, such as the 20:4 or the one meal a day (OMAD) protocol, a midday workout may be more suitable. This allows you to exercise during the later stages of your fast when fat burning is at its peak.
- Evening workouts: For some, evening workouts feel most comfortable, especially if they coincide with the end of their fasting window. This timing can help ensure that your body is refueled with nutrients post-workout, promoting recovery and muscle growth.

2. Listen to Your Body

As you experiment with different workout timings, it's essential to listen to your body and pay attention to how you feel. If you find that a specific time leaves you feeling drained or lightheaded, consider adjusting your workout schedule or modifying the intensity of your exercise.

3. Fueling and Refueling

Regardless of when you choose to work out, it's essential to fuel your body properly before and after exercise. During your eating window, focus on consuming nutrient-dense foods that provide a balance of protein, carbohydrates, and healthy fats. This will ensure that your body has the necessary fuel for your workouts and the nutrients required for recovery and muscle growth.

Finding the optimal timing for your workouts during intermittent fasting can take some trial and error, but it's worth the effort.

By paying attention to your body's signals and experimenting with different workout times, you can find a schedule that works best for your unique needs and goals.

Ultimately, the key is to be flexible, adaptable, and open to making adjustments as you progress on your fitness journey.

Chapter 6: Common Challenges and Solutions

Overcoming Hunger Pangs

One of the most common difficulties people face when starting IF is dealing with hunger pangs. In this chapter, we will explore various strategies to help you manage and overcome this problem as you incorporate IF into your daily routine.

A. **Understanding Hunger Pangs**

Before we delve into the solutions, it's crucial to understand what hunger pangs are and why they occur. Hunger pangs, also known as hunger pains, are physical sensations of discomfort, gnawing, or emptiness in the stomach, usually accompanied by the desire to eat.

They can be triggered by various factors, such as low blood sugar levels, hormonal fluctuations, or the body's natural response to an empty stomach.

B. **Stay Hydrated**

Drinking water is a simple yet effective way to manage hunger pangs. Water takes up space in your stomach, making you feel full and reducing the sensation of hunger. Additionally, thirst is often mistaken for hunger, so staying hydrated can help prevent unnecessary eating.

Aim to drink at least 8-10 glasses of water per day and consider sipping on herbal teas or black coffee during your fasting window. Just be sure to avoid sweeteners and high-calorie beverages, which could break your fast.

C. Consume Fiber-Rich Foods

Fiber is an essential component of a well-rounded diet and can be particularly helpful in combating hunger pangs. Foods high in fiber, such as fruits, vegetables, whole grains, and legumes, can increase satiety and keep you feeling fuller for longer periods. Incorporating these foods into your eating window can help you stay satisfied and maintain energy levels throughout your fasting period.

D. Balance Your Macronutrients

A balanced macronutrient intake – consisting of carbohydrates, proteins, and fats – is essential for maintaining stable blood sugar levels and preventing excessive hunger. Ensure that your meals are well-rounded, with adequate amounts of healthy fats, lean protein, and complex carbohydrates. This balance can help you stay satiated and support your body's nutritional needs during your fasting window.

E. Practice Mindful Eating

Mindful eating is the practice of being fully present and aware of the eating experience. This approach encourages you to pay attention to your body's hunger and fullness cues, helping you differentiate between physical hunger and emotional or habitual eating. By becoming more in tune with your body's signals, you can better manage hunger pangs during your fasting window.

F. **Distract Yourself**

Sometimes, hunger pangs are more psychological than physiological. When you're used to eating at specific times or as a response to certain situations, hunger pangs may appear out of habit rather than actual need. In these cases, engaging in activities that keep your mind occupied can help you ride out the hunger wave. Try going for a walk, reading a book, or immersing yourself in a hobby to take your focus away from food.

G. **Gradually Increase Fasting Duration**

If you're new to IF, jumping straight into longer fasting windows might be overwhelming for your body. Instead, consider gradually increasing your fasting duration to give your body time to adapt. Start with shorter fasting periods and then incrementally lengthen them as you become more comfortable with the practice.

H. **Be Patient and Persistent**

Lastly, it's essential to remember that adapting to IF takes time, and hunger pangs are a normal part of the adjustment process. Be patient with yourself and stay committed to your goals. Over time, your body will adapt, and managing hunger pangs will become easier.

Dealing with hunger pangs is a common challenge for those beginning an intermittent fasting journey. However, by understanding the causes of hunger pangs and employing strategies such as staying hydrated, consuming fiber-rich foods, balancing macronutrients, practicing mindful eating, distracting yourself, gradually increasing fasting duration, and being patient, you can overcome this hurdle and successfully incorporate IF into your lifestyle.

As you progress in your IF journey, you'll find that your body becomes more accustomed to the fasting periods, and hunger pangs will likely diminish in intensity and frequency.
Remember that it's crucial to listen to your body and adjust your fasting routine accordingly. Don't be afraid to experiment with different fasting schedules or protocols to find the one that best suits your needs and lifestyle.

In the following sections, we will continue to explore other common challenges associated with intermittent fasting and provide practical solutions to help you succeed in your health goals.

By addressing these challenges head-on and implementing the strategies outlined in this book, you'll be well on your way to enjoying the many benefits of intermittent fasting, including improved weight management, increased energy levels, and overall enhanced well-being.

Dealing with Social and Family Pressure

When embarking on an intermittent fasting journey, one of the major challenges you may face is dealing with social and family pressure. While you've made a well-informed decision based on your health goals, it's important to remember that your friends and family may not fully understand your choices. In this chapter, we'll explore strategies to help you navigate these interactions while maintaining your commitment to intermittent fasting.

1. Educate and Inform

The first step in dealing with social and family pressure is to educate those around you about intermittent fasting. Many people hold misconceptions about this practice, often stemming from a lack of understanding. Share your reasons for adopting intermittent fasting, the science behind it, and the benefits you've experienced so far. By providing accurate information, you can help dispel any myths or concerns.

2. Be Patient and Respectful

As you share your new lifestyle choice, remember to be patient and respectful towards the opinions of others. Not everyone will be immediately supportive or understanding, and that's okay. Keep in mind that people have different perspectives, and it's not your responsibility to convince them. Instead, focus on maintaining a respectful dialogue and answering any questions they may have.

3. Set Boundaries

While it's important to be open and understanding, it's also crucial to set boundaries. Clearly communicate your fasting schedule and let your friends and family know that you won't be participating in certain activities during your fasting window. By being upfront about your limitations, you can avoid potential conflicts and misunderstandings.

4. Offer Alternative Ways to Socialize

Food often plays a central role in social gatherings, but it doesn't have to be the main focus. Suggest alternative ways to spend time together that don't revolve around food, such as going for a walk, attending a fitness class, or exploring a new hobby. This allows you to maintain social connections while sticking to your fasting schedule.

5. Bring Your Own Food or Snacks

In some social situations, it might be difficult to find suitable options that align with your fasting plan. To avoid this, consider bringing your own food or snacks to gatherings. This can help you stay on track while still enjoying the company of your friends and family. Let your host know in advance about your dietary needs, so they are not caught off guard.

6. Be Flexible and Plan Ahead

There will be times when you may need to adjust your fasting schedule to accommodate social events or family gatherings. When possible, plan ahead and shift your fasting window accordingly. Remember that intermittent fasting is meant to be a flexible lifestyle, and it's okay to make occasional adjustments to maintain balance in your life.

7. **Find Support**

Connecting with others who practice intermittent fasting can be incredibly beneficial. Reach out to online forums, social media groups, or local meetups to find like-minded individuals who can provide advice, encouragement, and understanding. Having a supportive network can make it easier to navigate social and family pressure.

8. **Embrace the Opportunity to Inspire**

Your dedication to intermittent fasting may inspire others to make positive changes in their own lives. Be open to sharing your experiences, and consider your journey as an opportunity to promote healthier habits. You may find that your friends and family become more supportive over time as they witness the positive impact it has on your life.

9. **Focus on Non-Food Activities**

Shift the focus of social gatherings from food to other enjoyable activities. Propose activities like game nights, movie nights, or outdoor adventures that don't revolve around food. This will help you avoid any awkward situations where you may feel pressured to eat outside of your eating window.

Dealing with social and family pressure while practicing intermittent fasting can be challenging. However, by educating others, setting boundaries, and maintaining a flexible mindset, you can successfully navigate these interactions.

Remember that you're making a conscious choice to prioritize your health, and that's something to be proud of. Stay true to your goals, and embrace the opportunity to inspire and support others along the way.

Managing Energy Levels

One of the most common challenges faced by individuals who adopt this dietary approach is managing their energy levels. Now we'll look at the reasons behind fluctuations in energy levels and provide practical tips to help you maintain a consistent energy flow during your fasting journey.

1. Understanding the body's energy sources

When you consume food, your body breaks it down into its basic components, including carbohydrates, proteins, and fats. These macronutrients are then converted into energy through various metabolic pathways.

Carbohydrates are the body's preferred source of energy, and they are broken down into glucose, which is used immediately or stored as glycogen in the liver and muscles. When you practice intermittent fasting, your body starts to deplete these glycogen stores, leading to a temporary drop in energy levels.

To maintain energy levels during fasting periods, the body switches to alternative energy sources, such as fat stores. This process, known as ketosis, results in the production of ketones, which can be used as a fuel source in the absence of carbohydrates.

2. Dealing with the initial energy dip

During the first few days of intermittent fasting, you may experience a decrease in energy levels as your body adjusts to the new eating schedule. This temporary dip can be attributed to the depletion of glycogen stores and the transition to ketosis. To help mitigate this initial energy slump, consider the following strategies:

- Gradually ease into intermittent fasting: Start by shortening your eating window by an hour or two and progressively increase the fasting duration over time. This gradual approach allows your body to adapt more easily to the new eating pattern.
- Stay hydrated: Drinking water throughout the day can help alleviate fatigue and maintain energy levels. You can also consume calorie-free beverages, such as black coffee or tea, during your fasting window to stay alert.
- Prioritize sleep: Ensure that you get enough rest at night, as sleep plays a critical role in maintaining energy levels and overall well-being.

3. **Maintaining energy levels in the long run**

Once you've adapted to intermittent fasting, you can take additional steps to maintain consistent energy levels:

- Balance your macronutrient intake: Consuming an appropriate balance of carbohydrates, proteins, and fats can help ensure that your body has the necessary nutrients to maintain energy levels. Consider consulting a nutritionist or using a macronutrient calculator to determine the ideal ratio for your specific needs.
- Focus on nutrient-dense foods: Choose whole foods rich in vitamins, minerals, and fiber to support your energy levels. Opt for lean proteins, whole grains, healthy fats, and plenty of fruits and vegetables during your eating window.
- Exercise regularly: Physical activity can help regulate blood sugar levels, improve insulin sensitivity, and boost your energy. However, avoid overly strenuous workouts during your fasting window, as this may lead to fatigue.
- Listen to your body: If you consistently feel low on energy or experience other adverse symptoms, it may be necessary to adjust your fasting protocol. Experiment with different fasting durations and eating windows to find the right balance for your body.

Managing energy levels while practicing intermittent fasting is crucial for long-term success. By understanding the body's energy sources and implementing practical strategies, you can maintain consistent energy levels and reap the full benefits of intermittent fasting.

Stay patient during the initial adaptation phase, prioritize self-care, and make adjustments as needed to create a sustainable fasting routine that works for you.

Chapter 7: Intermittent Fasting for Specific Populations

Fasting for Women: Hormonal Considerations

It's essential to recognize that women have unique hormonal considerations that must be taken into account when embarking on an intermittent fasting journey, so let's look into the specific concerns related to fasting for women and provide guidance on how to navigate these challenges for optimal results.

The Role of Hormones

Before diving into the intricacies of intermittent fasting for women, it's crucial to understand the role hormones play in our overall health. Hormones are chemical messengers that regulate various processes in the body, such as growth, metabolism, mood, and reproduction.

Women's hormonal health is a delicate balance, and any disruption to this equilibrium can result in a myriad of issues, including irregular menstrual cycles, mood swings, and hormonal imbalances.

Key Hormones Affected by Fasting

Two primary hormones that are influenced by intermittent fasting in women are estrogen and progesterone. Estrogen is responsible for regulating the menstrual cycle and maintaining bone density, while progesterone is essential for maintaining a healthy pregnancy and balancing the effects of estrogen. When fasting, fluctuations in these hormone levels can occur, which can lead to changes in menstrual regularity, mood, and energy levels.

Leptin and ghrelin, the hormones responsible for regulating hunger and satiety, are also impacted by fasting. Leptin levels decrease during fasting, which can lead to increased hunger, while ghrelin levels rise, resulting in a heightened sense of fullness.

Balancing these hormones is key for successful weight management and overall well-being.

Fasting Strategies for Women
With hormonal considerations in mind, it's crucial to approach intermittent fasting with a tailored strategy that accounts for individual needs and preferences. Here are some strategies to consider:

1. Gradual introduction: Instead of diving headfirst into a strict fasting regimen, start with a more gentle approach. For instance, try a 12-hour fasting window (such as 7 a.m. to 7 p.m.) for a few weeks, then slowly increase the fasting window as your body becomes accustomed to the changes.
2. Cycle syncing: Align your fasting schedule with your menstrual cycle to support hormonal balance. For example, during the follicular phase (the first half of your cycle), opt for a more extended fasting window,

such as 16:8. In the luteal phase (the second half of your cycle), switch to a shorter fasting window, like 12:12, to prevent hormonal imbalances.

3. Monitor your body: Keep track of how your body responds to intermittent fasting. If you notice any irregularities in your menstrual cycle or experience mood swings, fatigue, or other adverse side effects, consider adjusting your fasting schedule or consulting with a healthcare professional.

4. Nutrient-dense meals: Prioritize nutrient-rich foods during your eating window, focusing on healthy fats, high-quality proteins, and plenty of vegetables. Adequate nutrition is essential for maintaining hormonal balance, particularly when fasting.

5. Listen to your body: Finally, remember that every woman is unique, and what works for one person may not be the best approach for another. Pay attention to your body's signals and be willing to modify your fasting plan as needed.

Intermittent fasting can be a powerful tool for women when tailored to account for hormonal considerations. By incorporating the strategies outlined in this chapter, you can optimize your fasting experience while maintaining hormonal balance and supporting overall health.

Intermittent Fasting for Seniors

As we age, our bodies undergo numerous changes, and it's essential to adjust our lifestyles to maintain optimal health.

Potential Benefits of Intermittent Fasting for Seniors

1. Weight management: As we age, our metabolism slows down, and weight gain becomes a common concern. Intermittent fasting can help regulate body weight by reducing overall calorie intake and promoting fat loss while preserving lean muscle mass.

2. Improved insulin sensitivity: Insulin resistance increases with age, leading to an elevated risk of type 2 diabetes. IF has been shown to improve insulin sensitivity, thus reducing the risk of developing diabetes.

3. Enhanced cognitive function: Some research suggests that intermittent fasting may help protect against age-related cognitive decline, as it promotes the production of brain-derived neurotrophic factor (BDNF), a protein essential for learning and memory.

4. Cellular repair and autophagy: Fasting triggers a process called autophagy, where cells break down and recycle damaged components. This cellular "housekeeping" is essential for maintaining optimal

cellular function and may help slow down the aging process.

5. Reduced inflammation: Chronic inflammation contributes to various age-related diseases. Intermittent fasting has been shown to reduce inflammation markers, potentially lowering the risk of diseases such as cardiovascular disease and arthritis.

Safety Considerations for Seniors

While intermittent fasting can offer numerous health benefits, it's essential to consider potential risks and adjustments for seniors:

1. Nutrient intake: As we age, our nutritional needs change, and it's crucial to ensure adequate nutrient intake during the eating window. Seniors should prioritize nutrient-dense foods such as fruits, vegetables, lean proteins, whole grains, and healthy fats.

2. Medication adjustments: Some medications, such as those for diabetes or blood pressure, may need to be adjusted when practicing IF. It's essential to consult your healthcare provider before starting an intermittent fasting regimen.

3. Risk of dehydration: Seniors are more susceptible to dehydration, and fasting periods may exacerbate this risk. Remember to drink plenty of water during both fasting and eating windows to stay hydrated.

4. Energy levels: Seniors may experience decreased energy levels during fasting periods. It's essential to listen to your body and adjust your fasting schedule

accordingly, perhaps starting with shorter fasting windows and gradually increasing them as you become more comfortable.

5. Pre-existing medical conditions: Seniors with pre-existing medical conditions, such as diabetes, kidney disease, or a history of eating disorders, should consult their healthcare provider before beginning intermittent fasting.

How to Get Started

If you're considering trying intermittent fasting as a senior, follow these steps to ensure a safe and effective experience:

1. Consult your healthcare provider: Discuss your interest in intermittent fasting with your healthcare provider to determine if it's appropriate for your specific health needs.

2. Choose a method: Select an IF method that fits your lifestyle and preferences. The 16/8 method is often the easiest for beginners, as it allows for a more extended eating window.

3. Plan your meals: Focus on nutrient-dense foods during your eating window to ensure you're meeting your nutritional needs. Plan your meals in advance, emphasizing a variety of fruits, vegetables, lean proteins, whole grains, and healthy fats.

4. Stay hydrated: Drink plenty of water throughout the day, both during fasting and eating windows, to prevent dehydration. Herbal teas and black coffee (without added sugar or cream) can also be consumed during fasting periods, as they contain minimal calories.

5. Listen to your body: Pay attention to how your body responds to fasting. If you feel weak or dizzy, consider shortening your fasting window or adjusting your eating schedule. Remember that it may take some time for your body to adapt to intermittent fasting.

6. Monitor your progress: Keep track of your health markers, such as weight, blood pressure, and blood sugar levels, to assess the effectiveness of your intermittent fasting regimen. Regular check-ups with your healthcare provider can also help ensure you're on the right track.

7. Be patient: Intermittent fasting is not a quick fix, and it may take time to see noticeable results. Be patient and give your body time to adjust to this new eating pattern.

Intermittent fasting can be a powerful tool for seniors looking to improve their health and well-being. By carefully considering safety factors and working closely with your healthcare provider, you can successfully incorporate intermittent fasting into your lifestyle.

Remember that consistency is key, and it's essential to find a fasting method that works best for your individual needs and preferences. With patience and dedication, you'll be on your way to reaping the many health benefits that intermittent fasting has to offer.

Fasting for Athletes and Bodybuilders

While many people use intermittent fasting to lose weight or maintain a healthy lifestyle, athletes and bodybuilders are also turning to this method to enhance their performance and results.

Benefits of Fasting for Athletes and Bodybuilders

1. Improved Body Composition

One of the most notable benefits of intermittent fasting for athletes and bodybuilders is its effect on body composition. Fasting can help reduce body fat while maintaining or even increasing lean muscle mass. This is particularly beneficial for those looking to achieve a more defined and sculpted physique.

2. Enhanced Recovery and Reduced Inflammation

Intermittent fasting has been shown to improve recovery and reduce inflammation. By allowing your body to take periodic breaks from digesting food, it can better focus on repairing damaged tissues and reducing inflammation. This can lead to faster recovery times and improved performance in the gym or on the field.

3. Increased Growth Hormone Production

Growth hormone is essential for muscle growth, recovery, and overall athletic performance. Research has shown that intermittent fasting can increase the production of growth hormone, leading to greater muscle gains and improved performance.

4. Improved Insulin Sensitivity

Intermittent fasting can improve insulin sensitivity, which is crucial for nutrient absorption and overall health. Improved insulin sensitivity allows your body to better utilize carbohydrates for energy, rather than storing them as fat. This can lead to better performance and more effective muscle-building.

Challenges and Considerations

While there are many benefits to incorporating intermittent fasting into your athletic or bodybuilding routine, it's essential to be aware of potential challenges.

1. Balancing Nutrient Intake

One of the main concerns for athletes and bodybuilders is ensuring that they consume enough nutrients to fuel their performance and recovery. Intermittent fasting can make this more challenging, as you have a limited window to consume your daily calories and macronutrients. Planning your meals and tracking your intake becomes even more critical when fasting to ensure you're getting the nutrients you need.

2. Performance During Fasting Windows

Some athletes may experience a dip in performance during their fasting window, as their body adjusts to functioning without a constant supply of food. It's essential to listen to your body and adjust your training intensity as needed. You may also want to schedule your workouts around your feeding window to ensure you have adequate fuel for high-intensity training sessions.

Best Practices for Fasting Athletes and Bodybuilders

1. Choose the Right Fasting Protocol

There are various intermittent fasting protocols, such as the 16/8 method, 5:2 method, and alternate-day fasting. It's essential to choose the one that best fits your training schedule and individual needs. Some athletes may prefer a daily fasting window, while others may benefit from fasting on rest days.

2. Prioritize Protein

Protein is crucial for muscle repair, growth, and recovery. Be sure to consume enough protein during your feeding window to support your athletic and bodybuilding goals. This may mean consuming larger protein-rich meals or incorporating protein shakes to meet your daily requirements.

3. Stay Hydrated

Staying hydrated is essential for overall health and performance, especially when fasting. Make sure to drink plenty of water throughout the day, including during your fasting window.

4. Monitor Your Progress and Adjust as Needed

As with any training or nutrition plan, it's crucial to monitor your progress and make adjustments as needed.

5. Ease into Fasting

If you're new to intermittent fasting, it's essential to ease into it gradually. Start with shorter fasting windows and progressively increase the duration over time. This will allow your body to adapt to the changes and help you better manage potential side effects, such as hunger or decreased energy levels.

6. Optimize Your Pre- and Post-Workout Nutrition

To maximize performance and recovery, be mindful of your pre- and post-workout nutrition. Try to schedule your workouts around your feeding window, so you have the energy needed for high-intensity sessions. Consuming a meal rich in carbohydrates and protein within an hour after your workout can help with muscle recovery and glycogen replenishment.

7. Listen to Your Body

Intermittent fasting can be an excellent tool for athletes and bodybuilders when done correctly. However, it's crucial to listen to your body and make adjustments as needed. If you find that fasting negatively impacts your performance or recovery, consider modifying your fasting protocol or discontinuing it altogether.

8. Consult with a Professional

Before starting any new nutrition or training program, it's always a good idea to consult with a professional, such as a sports nutritionist or a certified personal trainer. They can help you tailor an intermittent fasting plan to your specific needs and goals, as well as provide guidance and support throughout the process.

Intermittent fasting can offer numerous benefits for athletes and bodybuilders, including improved body composition, enhanced recovery, and increased growth hormone production.

However, it's essential to approach fasting mindfully, choose the right protocol, and prioritize proper nutrition. By doing so, you can effectively incorporate intermittent fasting into your training regimen and enjoy the benefits it has to offer.

Fasting with Medical Conditions: Precautions and Contraindications

In this section, we'll explore the precautions and contraindications of intermittent fasting for individuals with specific medical conditions.

Before we delve into the specifics, it's important to note that this chapter is not intended as medical advice. Always consult with a qualified healthcare professional before making significant changes to your diet or lifestyle, especially if you have an existing medical condition.

1. Diabetes

Diabetes is a chronic condition in which the body either does not produce enough insulin or is unable to effectively use the insulin it produces. For those with diabetes, it's crucial to maintain stable blood sugar levels, and fasting can sometimes create complications.

For individuals with type 1 diabetes, intermittent fasting is generally not recommended. The risk of hypoglycemia (low blood sugar) is high, and it can be life-threatening if not managed properly. If you have type 1 diabetes and are considering fasting, consult with your healthcare provider and be prepared for close monitoring and adjustments to your insulin regimen.

People with type 2 diabetes should also approach intermittent fasting with caution. Some studies have shown that intermittent fasting may help improve blood sugar control, insulin sensitivity, and weight loss in individuals with type 2 diabetes. However, these potential benefits must be weighed against the risk of hypoglycemia. Always work closely with your healthcare provider to ensure that fasting is safe and appropriate for your specific situation.

2. Eating Disorders

For individuals with a history of eating disorders, such as anorexia nervosa, bulimia nervosa, or binge eating disorder, intermittent fasting may not be a suitable dietary approach. The restrictive nature of fasting can exacerbate disordered eating patterns and trigger negative thoughts or behaviors around food.

If you have a history of eating disorders or are currently struggling with one, it's crucial to prioritize your mental health and seek guidance from a qualified professional before attempting any form of fasting.

3. Pregnancy and Breastfeeding

Pregnancy and breastfeeding are times of increased nutritional demands, as both mother and baby require adequate nutrients for optimal growth and development. Intermittent fasting during pregnancy or while breastfeeding is generally not recommended, as it may compromise the intake of essential nutrients and negatively impact the health of both mother and baby.

4. Malnutrition and Underweight

If you are underweight or malnourished, intermittent fasting may not be the best choice for you. Fasting can exacerbate nutritional deficiencies and further compromise your health. Instead, focus on consuming a nutrient-dense, balanced diet to support your body's needs and promote overall health.

5. Certain Medications

Some medications, such as those for blood pressure or heart conditions, may require you to take them with food. Intermittent fasting may affect the absorption and effectiveness of these medications, making it crucial to discuss your intentions with your healthcare provider before beginning a fasting regimen.

6. Chronic Kidney Disease

Individuals with chronic kidney disease (CKD) should approach intermittent fasting with caution. Fasting may increase the risk of dehydration, electrolyte imbalances, and acidosis in those with CKD, potentially leading to further kidney damage. It's essential to consult with a nephrologist or renal dietitian before attempting intermittent fasting if you have kidney disease.

7. Thyroid Disorders

People with thyroid disorders, such as hypothyroidism or hyperthyroidism, should be cautious when considering intermittent fasting. The thyroid gland is responsible for regulating metabolism, and fasting may cause fluctuations in hormone levels that can exacerbate existing thyroid issues. Consult with your healthcare provider and closely monitor your thyroid hormone levels if you decide to experiment with intermittent fasting.

8. Adrenal Fatigue

Adrenal fatigue, also known as adrenal insufficiency, occurs when the adrenal glands cannot produce sufficient amounts of stress hormones, such as cortisol. Intermittent fasting may cause additional stress on the body, potentially worsening adrenal fatigue. If you suffer from adrenal fatigue or any form of adrenal insufficiency, consult with your healthcare provider before attempting fasting.

9. Autoimmune Conditions

Individuals with autoimmune conditions, such as rheumatoid arthritis, lupus, or multiple sclerosis, may experience varying effects from intermittent fasting. While some studies suggest that fasting can help reduce inflammation and improve immune function, others indicate that fasting may exacerbate certain autoimmune symptoms. It's crucial to work with your healthcare provider to monitor your condition and determine whether fasting is appropriate for you.

The bottom line is that intermittent fasting is not a one-size-fits-all approach. It's essential to understand your unique health circumstances and work closely with your healthcare provider to determine whether fasting is right for you.

By taking a personalized approach to fasting, you can optimize your health and well-being while minimizing potential risks.

Chapter 8: Measuring and Tracking Your Progress

Setting Realistic Goals

Although intermittent fasting is a versatile and customizable approach to eating, to successfully implement intermittent fasting into your life, it's crucial to set realistic goals and track your progress.

Before diving into the world of intermittent fasting, you must first understand your motivations and reasons for choosing this approach. Consider your health goals, such as weight loss, improved focus, or better blood sugar control.

Understanding your "why" will help you stay committed and set realistic expectations for your journey.
When setting goals, it's essential to make them SMART: Specific, Measurable, Achievable, Relevant, and Time-bound.

Here's how to apply these principles to intermittent fasting:

1. Specific: Be clear about what you want to achieve. Instead of setting a vague goal like "losing weight," specify the amount of weight you'd like to lose (e.g., 10 pounds) or a desired body fat percentage.

2. Measurable: Ensure that your goals can be tracked and measured. For example, if your goal is to improve blood sugar control, you can monitor your fasting blood glucose levels or HbA1c values.

3. Achievable: Set realistic and attainable goals based on your current situation and capabilities. If you're new to intermittent fasting, it's better to start with a less restrictive eating window (e.g., 14:10) and gradually work your way up to a more challenging fasting schedule.

4. Relevant: Your goals should align with your overall health and wellness objectives. For example, if you're aiming for better cardiovascular health, you might want to focus on improving your blood lipid profile and blood pressure readings.

5. Time-bound: Set a deadline for achieving your goals. This will help you stay focused and motivated. For example, you could set a goal of losing 10 pounds within the next three months.

Once you've established your SMART goals, it's time to track your progress. There are several ways to do this, and you can choose the method that works best for you.
Some options include:

- Keeping a food diary: Documenting your meals and fasting windows can help you stay accountable and make adjustments as needed.
- Monitoring body weight and measurements: Regularly checking your weight and taking body

measurements can provide tangible evidence of your progress.

- Logging blood markers: If you're tracking health markers such as blood glucose or cholesterol levels, record these values consistently to observe trends and improvements.
- Using mobile apps: Numerous smartphone apps can help you track your fasting windows, meals, and health metrics. Popular options include Zero, MyFitnessPal, and Life Fasting Tracker.

Remember, progress may not always be linear, and it's essential to stay patient and consistent. Don't be too hard on yourself if you experience setbacks or plateaus. Instead, use these experiences to learn and adjust your approach as needed.

As you continue your intermittent fasting journey, you'll gain valuable insights into your body and learn how to optimize your health and well-being.

Monitoring Weight Loss and Body Composition

As you embark on your journey with intermittent fasting, it's essential to monitor your progress to ensure you're achieving your desired results. Let's look at how to effectively track weight loss and body composition changes during intermittent fasting, and explore various methods and tools to help you assess your progress.

The Importance of Tracking Your Progress

Regularly monitoring your weight loss and body composition changes can help you stay motivated, maintain accountability, and make necessary adjustments to your intermittent fasting plan.

By keeping track of your progress, you will have a clearer understanding of how your body is responding to the intermittent fasting protocol and whether you need to make any modifications to achieve your goals.

Weight Loss vs. Fat Loss

When discussing weight loss, it's important to differentiate between losing weight and losing fat. While the numbers on the scale may decrease, this doesn't always equate to fat loss. You might be losing water weight or even lean muscle mass, which is not ideal. Tracking changes in your body composition, rather than just weight, will give you a more accurate picture of your progress.

Methods for Monitoring Weight Loss

1. Weighing Yourself: While it's not the most accurate measure of fat loss, weighing yourself regularly can still give you an idea of your overall progress. It's best to weigh yourself at the same time each day, preferably in the morning after using the bathroom and before eating or drinking. Keep in mind that daily fluctuations are normal, so it's essential to focus on trends over time rather than individual measurements.

2. Body Measurements: Taking body measurements can help you monitor changes in your body size and shape. Use a flexible tape measure to record the circumference of your waist, hips, thighs, and other areas of interest. Be consistent with your measurement technique and track changes over time.

3. Progress Photos: Visual documentation of your journey can be a powerful motivator. Take regular progress photos in the same lighting and poses to see how your body is changing. You may notice changes in your body that are not reflected in your weight or measurements.

Methods for Monitoring Body Composition

1. Skinfold Calipers: This method involves pinching the skin and fat layer at various points on your body and measuring the thickness with a caliper. While not as accurate as other methods, skinfold calipers can provide a relatively affordable and accessible way to track changes in body fat over time.

2. Bioelectrical Impedance Analysis (BIA): BIA devices send a small electrical current through your body to estimate body composition. These devices can range from affordable home scales to more expensive professional models. While not as accurate as other methods, BIA can provide a convenient way to track changes in body fat and lean mass.

3. Dual-Energy X-ray Absorptiometry (DEXA) Scan: DEXA scans use low-dose X-rays to provide highly

accurate measurements of body composition. However, this method can be expensive and may not be readily accessible to everyone.

4. Hydrostatic Weighing: Also known as underwater weighing, this method involves submerging yourself in water to measure body composition. While highly accurate, hydrostatic weighing is typically only available at specialized facilities and can be costly.

5. Air Displacement Plethysmography (Bod Pod): The Bod Pod uses air displacement to measure body composition. Similar in accuracy to hydrostatic weighing, this method is also usually only available at specialized facilities and can be expensive.

Tracking your weight loss and body composition changes during intermittent fasting is crucial for staying motivated and ensuring you achieve your desired results. By incorporating a combination of methods to monitor your progress, you'll be better equipped to make any necessary adjustments to your intermittent fasting plan and maintain a healthy, sustainable lifestyle.

Assessing Health Markers and Improvements

1. Body Composition: Weight and Body Fat Percentage

One of the most noticeable and easily measurable improvements brought on by intermittent fasting is a

change in body composition. Many people experience weight loss and a reduction in body fat percentage.
This can be attributed to a combination of factors, including reduced calorie intake, increased fat-burning, and the hormonal changes that occur during fasting.

To track these changes, you can use a body weight scale and a body fat measuring device, such as a bioelectrical impedance scale or skinfold calipers. It is essential to remember that your weight may fluctuate daily due to factors like hydration, so it's best to measure yourself at the same time every day, preferably in the morning.

2. Blood Sugar and Insulin Sensitivity

Intermittent fasting has been shown to improve blood sugar control and insulin sensitivity. This is crucial for preventing and managing type 2 diabetes, as well as maintaining overall metabolic health.
To track these improvements, you can use a blood glucose meter to measure your fasting blood sugar levels. Additionally, you can request a blood test from your healthcare provider to assess your HbA1c levels, which gives you an average of your blood sugar levels over the past three months.

3. Lipid Profile: Cholesterol and Triglycerides

Another key health marker impacted by intermittent fasting is your lipid profile, specifically your cholesterol and triglyceride levels. Research has shown that fasting can lead to improvements in high-density lipoprotein (HDL) cholesterol, also known as "good" cholesterol, and reductions in low-density lipoprotein (LDL) cholesterol and triglycerides.

To track these changes, request a lipid panel from your healthcare provider.

4. Blood Pressure

High blood pressure, or hypertension, is a major risk factor for cardiovascular disease. Intermittent fasting can help improve blood pressure by reducing inflammation, improving insulin sensitivity, and promoting weight loss. To track your blood pressure, invest in a home blood pressure monitor or visit your healthcare provider regularly.

5. Inflammation and Oxidative Stress

Inflammation and oxidative stress contribute to numerous chronic diseases and the aging process. Intermittent fasting can help reduce inflammation and oxidative stress by promoting cellular repair and autophagy, which is the body's process of cleaning out damaged cells and regenerating new ones.

To track these improvements, you can request blood tests for inflammatory markers, such as C-reactive protein (CRP), from your healthcare provider.

6. Cognitive Function and Mental Well-being

Intermittent fasting may also have positive effects on cognitive function and mental well-being. Research has shown that fasting can boost brain-derived neurotrophic factor (BDNF), which is essential for learning, memory, and mood regulation.

To assess improvements in cognitive function, pay attention to your ability to concentrate, your memory, and your overall mental clarity. For mental well-being, consider tracking your mood and energy levels.

7. Gut Health and Microbiome

Intermittent fasting may also have a positive impact on your gut health and microbiome. The gut microbiome plays a vital role in maintaining your immune system, digestion, and overall health. Fasting can help improve gut health by promoting a diverse and healthy microbiome and increasing the production of short-chain fatty acids (SCFAs), which are essential for maintaining gut barrier integrity.

To assess improvements in gut health, you can monitor symptoms related to digestion and request a comprehensive stool analysis from your healthcare provider.

8. Sleep Quality

Sleep is essential for optimal health and well-being. Intermittent fasting may help improve sleep quality by regulating hormones and promoting a healthy circadian rhythm.

To track your sleep improvements, consider using a sleep tracking app or device to monitor sleep duration, sleep stages, and overall sleep quality. Additionally, pay attention to how you feel upon waking and throughout the day, as better sleep often leads to increased energy levels and improved mood.

9. Physical Performance and Endurance

Intermittent fasting has the potential to improve physical performance and endurance by enhancing the body's ability to use stored fat as fuel, which can be particularly beneficial for endurance athletes.

To measure these improvements, track your exercise performance, such as the time it takes to complete a specific workout, the amount of weight you can lift, or the distance you can run. You may also want to consider using a heart rate monitor to assess your cardiovascular fitness.

10. Hormone Balance

Lastly, intermittent fasting can help balance hormones, such as insulin, human growth hormone (HGH), and leptin, which play crucial roles in metabolism, muscle growth, and appetite regulation.

To assess improvements in hormone balance, you can request blood tests from your healthcare provider to measure hormone levels.

By closely monitoring these health markers, you can gain valuable insights into the improvements that intermittent fasting brings to your overall health.

Remember that individual results will vary, and it's essential to consult with a healthcare professional before making significant changes to your diet or lifestyle.

Stay consistent, be patient, and track your progress to experience the transformative power of intermittent fasting on your health and well-being.

Chapter 9: Intermittent Fasting Myths and Misconceptions

Debunking Common Fasting Myths

Welcome to Chapter 9, where we dive into the myths and misconceptions surrounding intermittent fasting. As with any health trend, it's easy for misinformation to circulate, which can lead to confusion and misunderstandings. That's why it's essential to separate fact from fiction, to ensure you make well-informed decisions about your health.

In this chapter, we'll debunk some of the most common fasting myths and provide you with the knowledge you need to make informed choices about your fasting journey.

Myth 1: Intermittent fasting is just another fad diet
Intermittent fasting is often mistakenly lumped in with fad diets that promise quick fixes and dramatic results. However, intermittent fasting is not a diet in the traditional sense.

Rather, it is an eating pattern that focuses on when you eat, rather than what you eat. This approach has been practiced for centuries across various cultures and religions for both health and spiritual reasons.

Recent scientific studies have also shown that intermittent fasting can provide numerous health benefits, including improved insulin sensitivity, weight loss, increased mental clarity, and reduced inflammation. As a result, intermittent fasting is increasingly being recognized as a sustainable and beneficial lifestyle choice, rather than a short-term fad diet.

Myth 2: Intermittent fasting will cause muscle loss

One of the most common concerns about intermittent fasting is the fear of losing muscle mass. However, studies have shown that intermittent fasting can actually help preserve muscle mass while promoting fat loss.

When you fast, your body produces human growth hormone (HGH), which helps to maintain lean body mass and stimulate fat burning.

Additionally, intermittent fasting has been shown to increase the efficiency of your workouts, enabling you to build muscle more effectively. By ensuring you consume adequate protein and nutrients during your eating window, you can maintain and even build muscle while practicing intermittent fasting.

Myth 3: Intermittent fasting leads to nutrient deficiencies

Some people believe that intermittent fasting can cause nutrient deficiencies due to the limited eating window. However, this is not necessarily the case. As long as you consume a balanced and nutrient-dense diet during your eating window, you can meet your nutritional needs while fasting.

In fact, intermittent fasting can encourage healthier eating habits by prompting individuals to be more mindful about their food choices. When you have a limited eating window, you're more likely to prioritize nutrient-dense foods over empty calories. This can lead to an overall improvement in the quality of your diet and help you avoid deficiencies.

Myth 4: Intermittent fasting slows down your metabolism

A common misconception is that fasting will slow down your metabolism, making it harder to lose weight. However, research has shown that short-term fasting can actually boost your metabolism, as your body becomes more efficient at burning fat for fuel. This metabolic switch is known as ketosis and can help you lose weight and improve your overall health.

It's important to note that prolonged fasting or severe calorie restriction can indeed slow down your metabolism. However, the intermittent fasting protocols most people follow (such as the 16:8 or 5:2 methods) do not typically result in a significant drop in metabolism, as long as you consume enough calories and nutrients during your eating window.

As you progress through your fasting journey, always remember to listen to your body, make informed choices, and consult with a healthcare professional if you have any concerns or underlying health conditions.

Addressing Criticisms and Concerns

While many people have found success with IF, it is not without its critics. Let's have a look at some of the most common criticisms and concerns surrounding intermittent fasting, offering both scientific evidence and practical guidance to help you make informed decisions about whether IF is right for you.

1. "Intermittent fasting is just another fad diet."

One of the most frequent criticisms of intermittent fasting is that it's just another passing fad. However, it's important to recognize that IF is not a diet in the traditional sense, as it doesn't dictate what you should eat, but rather when you should eat. Moreover, fasting has been practiced for centuries across various cultures and religions, indicating that it is not merely a contemporary trend.

Recent scientific research supports the idea that intermittent fasting can provide significant health benefits, including weight loss, improved cardiovascular health, and increased insulin sensitivity. As more studies emerge, it's becoming clear that IF is not just a passing fad but a legitimate dietary strategy for many people.

2. "Intermittent fasting is too restrictive and difficult to maintain."

Some critics argue that the eating windows prescribed by intermittent fasting can be too restrictive and challenging to adhere to, particularly for those with busy schedules or social commitments. While it's true that IF can require discipline and planning, the flexibility of various IF protocols allows individuals to find an approach that works best for them.

For instance, there are several popular intermittent fasting methods, such as the 16/8 method (fasting for 16 hours and eating within an 8-hour window), the 5:2 method (consuming a normal diet for five days and restricting calories to 500-600 on two non-consecutive days), or alternate-day fasting. You can experiment with different methods to find a sustainable and enjoyable way to incorporate IF into your lifestyle.

3. "Intermittent fasting can lead to disordered eating and obsession with food."

There is a valid concern that intermittent fasting may encourage disordered eating patterns, particularly for individuals with a history of eating disorders. However, it's essential to differentiate between the controlled and intentional nature of IF and the chaotic, unhealthy patterns associated with disordered eating.

It's crucial for individuals considering IF to listen to their bodies, prioritize their mental health, and seek professional guidance if needed. If you find that IF is causing you to obsess over food or feel guilt and shame around eating, it may not be the right approach for you.

4. **"Intermittent fasting can cause muscle loss and negatively impact athletic performance."**

Some critics argue that IF can lead to muscle loss and decreased athletic performance. While it's true that fasting can cause the body to break down muscle tissue for energy, proper nutrition and exercise can help mitigate this effect. Incorporating adequate protein and strength training into your routine can help maintain muscle mass during periods of fasting. Additionally, some studies have shown that intermittent fasting can improve endurance and exercise efficiency, suggesting that, for some athletes, IF may not necessarily be detrimental to performance.

5. **"Intermittent fasting is not suitable for everyone."**

This criticism is valid, as intermittent fasting is not a one-size-fits-all approach. Certain populations, such as pregnant or breastfeeding women, growing children and teenagers, individuals with diabetes, or those with a history of disordered eating, may not be well-suited for IF. Before embarking on an intermittent fasting journey, it's essential to consult with a healthcare professional to determine whether this approach is appropriate for your unique circumstances.

While intermittent fasting may not be suitable for everyone, it is a legitimate and effective dietary strategy for many individuals. By addressing these common criticisms and concerns, we hope to provide you with a more comprehensive understanding of intermittent fasting and its potential benefits and drawbacks.

As with any lifestyle change, it's crucial to be mindful of your body's signals, prioritize your mental and physical well-being, and consult with a healthcare professional to ensure that intermittent fasting is the right choice for you. By doing so, you can make an informed decision about whether to incorporate IF into your life and potentially reap its numerous health benefits.

Remember that intermittent fasting is just one tool in the toolbox of health-promoting strategies. A balanced diet, regular exercise, stress management, and adequate sleep are equally important factors in maintaining overall health and well-being. Finding a sustainable and enjoyable approach to your nutrition and lifestyle habits is key to long-term success.

So, if you're considering intermittent fasting, take the time to carefully weigh the pros and cons, keeping in mind the various concerns and criticisms. Be patient with yourself as you experiment with different IF protocols, and don't hesitate to seek guidance from healthcare professionals or nutrition experts to ensure that your intermittent fasting journey is a safe and successful one.

Chapter 10: Your Intermittent Fasting Journey

Developing a Personalized Fasting Plan

Welcome to Chapter 10! By now, you've learned a lot about intermittent fasting, its benefits, and various methods.
Now it's time to start your own journey and develop a personalized fasting plan that suits your lifestyle, goals, and preferences.

Remember, there's no one-size-fits-all approach, so be ready to experiment and find what works best for you.

In this chapter, we'll cover the following topics:

    A. Understanding your goals
    B. Choosing the right fasting method
    C. Personalizing your eating window
    D. Adapting your plan to your lifestyle
    E. Monitoring progress and making adjustments

A. Understanding Your Goals

Before you start any new health regimen, it's crucial to understand your goals. Are you aiming to lose weight, improve your overall health, increase mental clarity, or all of the above? Knowing your goals will help you choose the right fasting method and duration, as well as help you track your progress.

Take some time to reflect on your goals and write them down. This will serve as a motivation and a reminder throughout your intermittent fasting journey.

B. **Choosing the Right Fasting Method**

As we've discussed in previous chapters, there are several intermittent fasting methods, including:

1. 16/8 method: Fasting for 16 hours and eating within an 8-hour window.
2. 5:2 method: Eating normally for five days and restricting calories for two non-consecutive days.
3. Eat-Stop-Eat: Fasting for 24 hours once or twice a week.
4. Alternate Day Fasting: Fasting every other day.

Choose a method that aligns with your goals, preferences, and lifestyle. If you're a beginner, you may want to start with a shorter fasting window, like the 16/8 method, and gradually work your way up as you become more comfortable with fasting. Keep in mind that it's always a good idea to consult with a healthcare professional before starting any new diet plan.

C. **Personalizing Your Eating Window**

Once you've chosen a fasting method, you'll need to decide when to eat and when to fast. The key here is to find a schedule that fits your daily routine and makes fasting feel as effortless as possible.

For instance, if you're a morning person who enjoys breakfast, consider adjusting your eating window to include breakfast and lunch, then fast through the evening and night. Conversely, if you're a night owl who prefers dinner, you may want to skip breakfast and start your eating window at lunchtime. Remember, there's no right or wrong way to do this – it's all about finding what works best for you.

D. **Adapting Your Plan to Your Lifestyle**

Intermittent fasting shouldn't feel like a punishment or an insurmountable challenge. Instead, it should be a sustainable and enjoyable part of your lifestyle. To ensure long-term success, consider the following tips:

1. Be flexible: Don't be afraid to adjust your fasting schedule to accommodate social events, work commitments, or other activities.
2. Stay hydrated: Drinking water during your fasting window can help stave off hunger and keep you feeling energized.
3. Make healthy food choices: Focus on nutrient-dense whole foods during your eating window, which will nourish your body and keep you feeling satisfied.
4. Prioritize sleep: Aim for 7-9 hours of quality sleep each night, as lack of sleep can affect your hunger hormones and make fasting more challenging.

E. **Monitoring Progress and Making Adjustments**

Once you've started your intermittent fasting journey, it's essential to track your progress and make adjustments as needed. Keep a journal to record your fasting schedule, food intake, energy levels, and any other relevant information. This will help you identify patterns, pinpoint potential issues, and make necessary adjustments to optimize your plan.

Additionally, consider tracking the following metrics to gauge your progress toward your goals:

1. Weight: While weight loss may not be your primary goal, it's essential to monitor it to ensure that you're not losing weight too rapidly or not at all.
2. Body composition: Use a body fat scale or calipers to measure your body fat percentage. This can help you understand whether you're losing fat or muscle mass, and make adjustments accordingly.
3. Blood markers: Regularly monitoring blood markers such as glucose, insulin, cholesterol, and inflammation can provide valuable insights into your overall health and the effectiveness of your fasting plan.
4. Subjective well-being: Pay attention to how you feel mentally and physically during your fasting journey. Are you feeling more energized, experiencing better mental clarity, or noticing improved sleep quality?

Remember, progress may not always be linear, and it's essential to be patient and give your body time to adjust. If you're not seeing the desired results or experiencing negative side effects, consider consulting with a healthcare professional for guidance.

Embarking on your intermittent fasting journey is an exciting and transformative experience. By developing a personalized fasting plan, you can maximize the benefits of intermittent fasting while minimizing potential challenges.

Stay open-minded, adaptable, and committed to your goals, and you'll be well on your way to a healthier and happier you!

Integrating Fasting into Your Lifestyle

Let's incorporate fasting into your daily routine and make it an enjoyable and sustainable part of your life.

1. **Understand the Types of Intermittent Fasting**

Before diving into the world of fasting, it's important to understand the various types of intermittent fasting methods. The most popular ones include:

- The 16/8 Method: This method involves fasting for 16 hours each day and eating all your meals within an 8-hour window. For example, you might skip breakfast and eat your first meal at noon and your last meal at 8 PM.

- The 5:2 Method: With this approach, you eat normally for five days a week and restrict your calorie intake to around 500-600 calories on the other two non-consecutive days.
- Eat-Stop-Eat: This method involves a 24-hour fast once or twice a week. You may choose to fast from breakfast to breakfast or from dinner to dinner, depending on your preferences.

Choose a method that best suits your lifestyle, goals, and personal preferences. Remember that intermittent fasting is meant to be a sustainable practice, so it's essential to find a method you can stick to in the long run.

2. Start Slowly and Gradually

If you're new to fasting, it's crucial to ease into it. Begin with shorter fasting periods, such as 12 hours, and gradually increase the duration as your body adapts. This will help minimize potential side effects like fatigue, irritability, and hunger pangs. Remember, it's a marathon, not a sprint – take your time to adjust and listen to your body.

3. Stay Hydrated

While fasting, it's essential to stay hydrated. Drinking water not only helps you feel full but also aids in flushing out toxins and supporting metabolic processes. You can also consume non-caloric beverages like black coffee, tea, and herbal infusions. However, be cautious about overdoing caffeinated drinks, as they may lead to restlessness and dehydration.

4. Plan Your Meals

Planning your meals during your eating window can make a significant difference in your fasting experience. Opt for nutrient-dense foods, such as whole grains, lean proteins, fruits, and vegetables, to ensure you're getting the necessary vitamins and minerals. Balanced meals will also help you feel satiated and maintain stable energy levels throughout the day.

5. Find Support

Having a support system can be invaluable when integrating fasting into your lifestyle. Connect with friends or family members who share your goals, or join online forums and social media groups dedicated to intermittent fasting. Sharing your experiences, challenges, and victories with like-minded individuals can help keep you motivated and accountable.

6. Be Flexible

Life is unpredictable, and it's essential to be flexible with your fasting schedule. Don't stress if you can't maintain your fasting window on a particular day due to social events, work commitments, or personal reasons. Simply resume your regular routine the following day. Remember that consistency over time is more important than perfection.

7. Monitor Your Progress

Keep track of your progress by regularly monitoring your weight, energy levels, and overall well-being. This can help you make adjustments to your fasting routine if necessary and will serve as a source of motivation when you see positive results.

8. Exercise Mindfully

Physical activity is an important aspect of overall health and can complement your fasting routine. However, it's crucial to listen to your body and adjust your exercise regimen accordingly. During the initial stages of fasting, you may need to reduce the intensity or duration of your workouts. As your body adapts to your new eating pattern, you can gradually increase the intensity of your exercise routine. Remember that balance is key, and overexerting yourself while fasting can be counterproductive.

9. Address Emotional Eating

Intermittent fasting can help you develop a healthier relationship with food by breaking the cycle of emotional eating. Take this opportunity to identify emotional triggers that may lead to overeating and learn healthier ways to cope with stress, anxiety, or boredom. Practicing mindfulness and meditation, engaging in hobbies, or seeking support from a therapist or counselor can help you better manage your emotions without relying on food.

10. Be Patient and Give Yourself Grace

Last but not least, be patient with yourself and give yourself grace as you embark on this journey. Integrating fasting into your lifestyle is a process that requires time, perseverance, and self-compassion. It's natural to experience setbacks and challenges along the way, but it's important to learn from them and keep moving forward. Celebrate your victories, no matter how small, and remember that your health and well-being are worth the effort.

By following these guidelines and adopting a positive and flexible mindset, you can successfully integrate fasting into your lifestyle and reap its numerous health benefits. Remember, the key to sustainable success lies in finding an approach that works best for you and supports your overall well-being.

Staying Motivated and Committed

Intermittent fasting, as with any lifestyle change, requires a certain level of dedication and motivation. Embarking on this journey can be challenging, but the long-term health benefits make it worth the effort.

Understand the "why" behind your decision Before diving into intermittent fasting, take the time to understand your reasons for choosing this lifestyle. Are you looking to improve your overall health, lose weight, or increase mental clarity? Knowing the "why" will help you stay focused and motivated during the tough times when temptation is high.

1. <u>Set realistic and achievable goals.</u> Setting specific, measurable, achievable, relevant, and time-bound (SMART) goals can help you stay motivated and committed to your intermittent fasting journey. For example, instead of setting a vague goal like "I want to lose weight," try something more specific, like "I want to lose 10 pounds in two months by practicing intermittent fasting and incorporating regular exercise." This way, you have a clear goal and a plan to achieve it.

2. <u>Track your progress.</u> Keep a journal or use an app to record your fasting hours, meals, and any changes you notice in your body and mind. By tracking your progress, you can celebrate your achievements and identify areas that may need improvement. Regularly reviewing your progress will help you stay accountable and motivated.

3. <u>Surround yourself with support.</u> Having a strong support system can make a significant difference in your intermittent fasting journey. Share your goals with friends, family, or join online communities of like-minded individuals. Engaging with others who are also practicing intermittent fasting can provide you with encouragement, tips, and valuable insights.

4. <u>Be flexible and adaptable.</u> Remember that everyone's intermittent fasting experience is different, and it's essential to listen to your body. If

you find that a specific fasting protocol isn't working for you, don't be afraid to modify your approach. Being open to change and adapting your plan can help you stay committed and prevent feelings of frustration or failure.

5. <u>Focus on the benefits.</u> When motivation wanes, remind yourself of the potential health benefits of intermittent fasting. These can include weight loss, improved insulin sensitivity, increased mental clarity, and better overall health. Keep these benefits at the forefront of your mind to stay motivated and committed.

6. <u>Celebrate your successes.</u> It's crucial to recognize and celebrate your achievements, no matter how small they may seem. Did you stick to your fasting schedule for a week without slipping up? Treat yourself to a relaxing bath or a new book. Acknowledging your hard work and success can help reinforce your commitment to intermittent fasting.

7. <u>Be patient.</u> Remember that change takes time, and it's normal to experience ups and downs throughout your intermittent fasting journey. It's essential to be patient with yourself and your progress. As you continue to practice intermittent fasting and make adjustments as needed, you'll likely see improvements in your health and well-being.

8. <u>Seek professional guidance if needed.</u> If you're struggling to stay motivated or need expert advice, consider seeking the guidance of a healthcare professional or nutritionist. They can help you

develop a personalized plan and provide valuable support throughout your journey.

Staying motivated and committed to intermittent fasting requires understanding your "why," setting realistic goals, tracking your progress, seeking support, being flexible, focusing on the benefits, celebrating your successes, being patient, and seeking professional guidance if needed. By adopting these strategies, you'll be better equipped to stay motivated and committed to your intermittent fasting journey, reaping the long-term health benefits it can provide.

Celebrating Success and Embracing Growth

Success Stories

Every journey begins with a single step, and in the world of intermittent fasting, countless individuals have taken that step and reaped the rewards.

These are people from all walks of life, each with their own unique challenges and goals, who have experienced remarkable transformations.

1. **The Weight Loss Winner:**
   Sarah, a 35-year-old mother of two, struggled with her weight for years. After trying various diets and workout regimens, she discovered intermittent fasting. Within six months of adopting a 16:8 fasting protocol (16 hours of fasting and an 8-hour eating

window), Sarah lost 45 pounds and regained her confidence. Her newfound energy allowed her to keep up with her kids and live life to the fullest.

2. **The Mental Clarity Champion:**
Mark, a 50-year-old entrepreneur, found it increasingly difficult to focus at work as he aged. Overwhelmed by stress and cognitive decline, Mark turned to intermittent fasting. By incorporating a 20:4 fasting protocol (20 hours of fasting and a 4-hour eating window), he noticed a significant improvement in his mental clarity and productivity, helping him make better business decisions and lead a more balanced life.

3. **The Health and Wellness Warrior:**
Jasmine, a 28-year-old fitness enthusiast, sought to improve her overall health and well-being. By adopting a 5:2 fasting protocol (eating normally for five days and restricting calories to 500-600 for two non-consecutive days), she noticed improvements in her sleep quality, digestion, and energy levels, enhancing her athletic performance and day-to-day life.

Embracing Growth

As with any lifestyle change, adopting intermittent fasting comes with its challenges. By acknowledging these challenges and learning from them, we can cultivate personal growth and make our fasting journey a fulfilling one.

1. Navigating Social Situations: One of the biggest challenges for intermittent fasters is managing social situations that revolve around food. Learn to communicate your dietary choices to others and remember that it's perfectly acceptable to participate in social events without consuming food. With practice, you'll become more confident and adept at navigating these situations.

2. Adjusting to Hunger Pangs: It's natural to feel hungry during the initial stages of intermittent fasting. As your body adjusts to this new eating pattern, hunger pangs will become less frequent and intense. Embrace this temporary discomfort as a sign of growth and focus on staying hydrated and consuming nutrient-dense foods during your eating window.

3. Overcoming Plateaus: It's not uncommon to hit a weight loss or fitness plateau while practicing intermittent fasting. This is an opportunity for growth and self-reflection. Reevaluate your fasting protocol, exercise routine, and food choices, and consider making adjustments to help you break through the plateau.

Intermittent fasting is way more than just a weight loss tool; it's a journey of personal growth and self-improvement.

By celebrating our successes, learning from our challenges, and embracing the growth that comes with change, we can create a healthier, happier, and more fulfilling life.

Chapter 11.
Conclusion/Summary/Final Thoughts

As we reach the end of our journey through the fascinating world of intermittent fasting, it's important to take a moment to reflect on what we've learned and how this powerful tool can be harnessed to improve our health and well-being.

Throughout this book, we've delved into the science, benefits, and practical aspects of intermittent fasting, and it's our hope that this knowledge has been both enlightening and inspiring.

Intermittent fasting is not a fad diet or a quick fix for weight loss. Rather, it's a lifestyle choice that has been practiced throughout human history and is now backed by an ever-growing body of scientific research.
By embracing intermittent fasting, you're not only tapping into the wisdom of our ancestors but also taking advantage of cutting-edge knowledge to optimize your health.

One of the key takeaways from our exploration of intermittent fasting is the variety of methods available. From the 16:8 approach to the 5:2 method, and from alternate-day fasting to the eat-stop-eat approach, there's a fasting regimen to suit just about every lifestyle and preference. This flexibility is one of the reasons intermittent fasting has become so popular and sustainable for many people.

We've also learned about the myriad health benefits associated with intermittent fasting. Beyond weight loss and improved body composition, fasting can help enhance mental clarity, increase energy levels, reduce inflammation, and even promote cellular repair and autophagy.

Furthermore, research has shown that intermittent fasting may help prevent or manage chronic conditions such as diabetes, heart disease, and even certain types of cancer.

It's important to remember, however, that intermittent fasting is not a one-size-fits-all solution, and individual results may vary. Some people may experience great success with a particular fasting protocol, while others may need to experiment and adjust their approach to find what works best for their body and lifestyle.

As with any major lifestyle change, it's crucial to listen to your body, seek guidance from a healthcare professional if needed, and be patient with the process.

Another essential aspect of intermittent fasting is the importance of maintaining a balanced and nutritious diet during your eating windows. Consuming nutrient-dense foods and staying well-hydrated are critical to ensuring that your body receives the fuel it needs to function optimally. Remember that intermittent fasting is not an excuse to overindulge in unhealthy foods or neglect proper nutrition.

We've also touched on some of the potential challenges and misconceptions associated with intermittent fasting. From hunger pangs to social pressure, adopting a fasting lifestyle may come with its fair share of hurdles.

By being prepared for these challenges and arming yourself with knowledge, you'll be better equipped to navigate them and stay on track with your fasting goals.

In conclusion, intermittent fasting is a powerful and adaptable tool that can offer a wide range of health benefits when practiced safely and consistently. By incorporating fasting into your lifestyle and making informed choices about your nutrition and overall well-being, you're taking a proactive step towards a healthier, happier, and more vibrant future.

As you continue on your journey with intermittent fasting, remember to stay curious, be open to learning and growth, and always prioritize your health and well-being.

Thank you for reading this book and I would like to take this opportunity to wish you health and happiness wherever you may go.

Intermittent fasting FAQ

1. ***What is intermittent fasting?***
    Intermittent fasting is an eating pattern that alternates between periods of eating and fasting.

2. ***How does it work?***
    During the fasting periods, typically lasting between 16-24 hours, the body is in a state of ketosis, in which it burns stored fat for energy instead of glucose from food.

3. ***What are the benefits?***
    Intermittent fasting is said to improve insulin sensitivity, promote weight loss, improve cardiovascular health, and even extend lifespan.

4. ***Are there any risks?***
    Some people may experience side effects such as headache, fatigue, and irritability during the fasting periods. It is not recommended for people with certain health conditions such as pregnant or breastfeeding women, diabetics, and those with a history of eating disorders.

5. ***Can I still exercise while fasting?***
    Yes, you can still exercise while fasting. In fact, some people find that they have more energy during the fasting period. It's important to listen to your body and adjust your routine as needed.

6. *Are there any foods I should avoid?*

There are no specific foods to avoid while intermittent fasting, but it's generally recommended to eat a healthy, balanced diet during the eating periods.

7. *How do I start?*

The easiest way to start is by choosing a 12- or 16-hour window for fasting, and gradually increasing the fasting period over time. Consult with a healthcare professional before starting any new diet or exercise program.

8. *Can I drink water while fasting?*

Yes, you can and should drink water while fasting. In fact, it's important to stay hydrated during the fasting period. Some people also drink non-caloric beverages such as black coffee or tea during the fasting period.

9. *Can I eat whatever I want during the eating periods?*

No, it's important to maintain a healthy, balanced diet during the eating periods. Eating a diet high in processed foods and added sugars can negate the benefits of intermittent fasting.

10. *Can I do intermittent fasting every day?*

Some people choose to do intermittent fasting every day, but it's also common to do it for certain days of the week or even just once or twice a week. It's important to listen to your body and adjust your routine as needed.

11. *Is it suitable for everyone?*

Intermittent fasting may not be suitable for everyone. It is not recommended for pregnant or breastfeeding women, diabetics, and those with a history of eating disorders. It's always a good idea to consult with a healthcare professional before starting any new diet or exercise program.

12. *How do I break a fast?*

When breaking a fast, it's important to ease back into eating. Start with small, easy-to-digest meals and gradually increase portion size. Avoid overeating and processed foods.

13. *Can I have a morning cup of tea or coffee when doing intermittent fasting?*

Yes, you can have a morning cup of tea or coffee while doing intermittent fasting, **BUT** it must be black tea or coffee because any beverage that contains calories, such as milk or sugar, will break the fast.

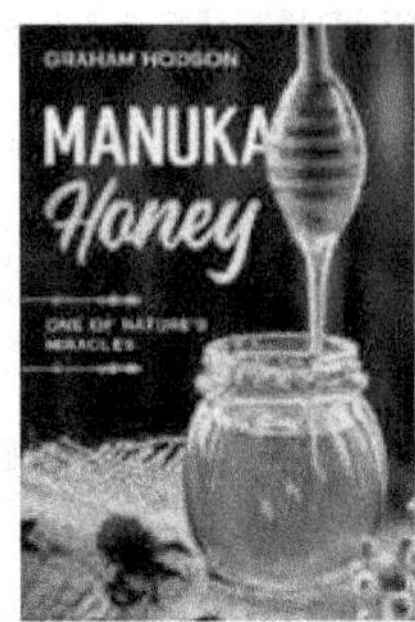
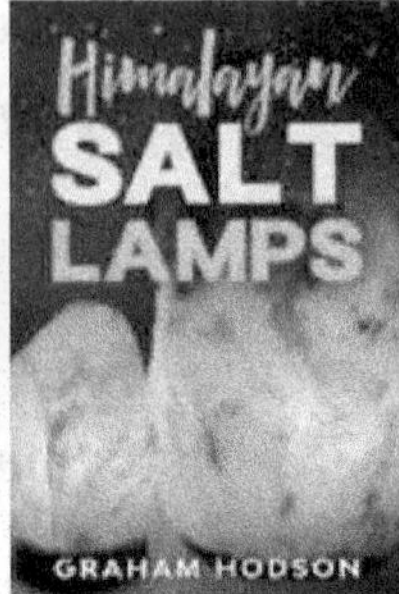
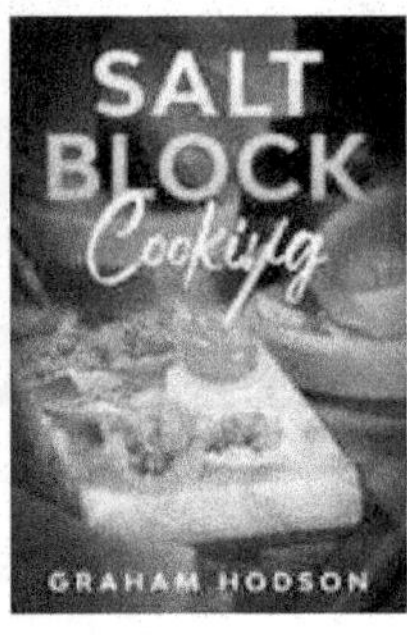
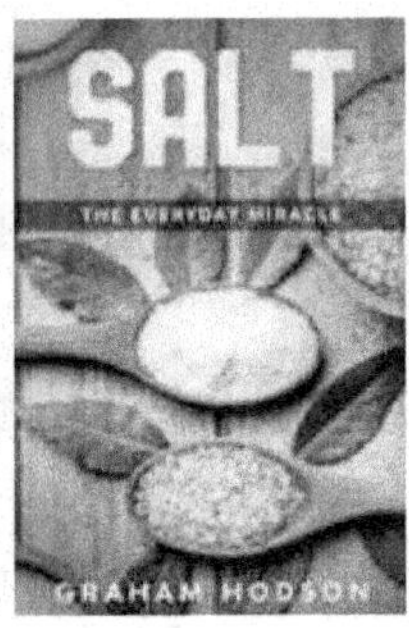
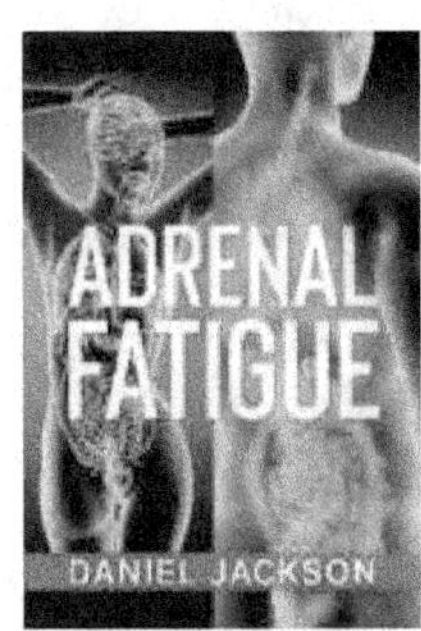
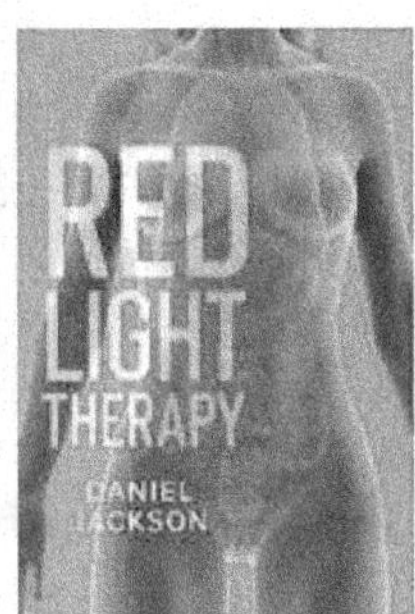
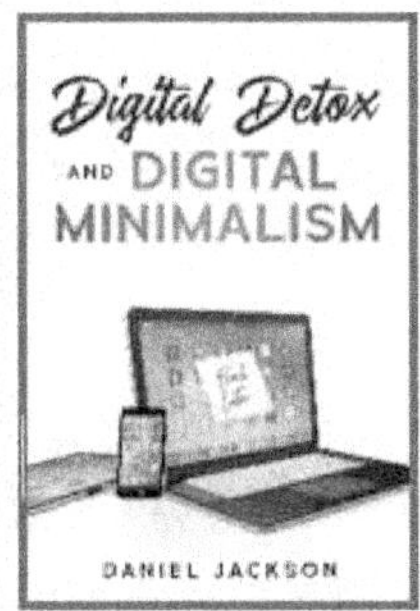
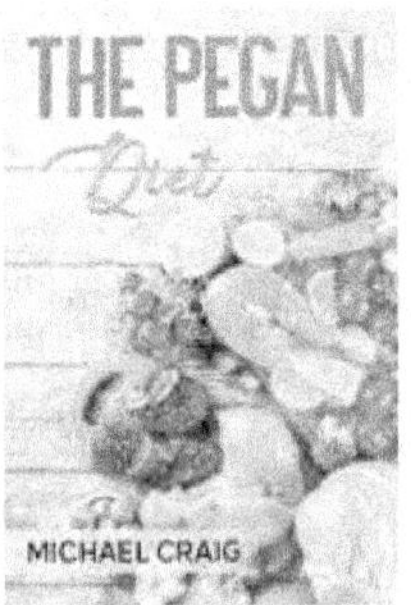

Take a look at more great books available from
Rockwood Publishing

… some for FREE!

Just visit the link below:

rockwoodpublishing.co.uk

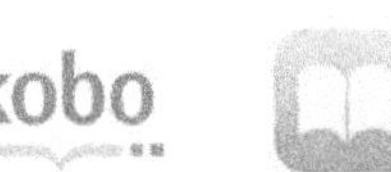
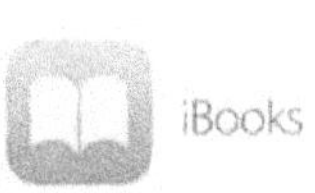
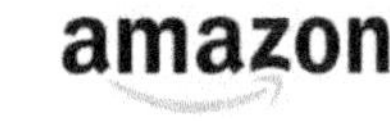
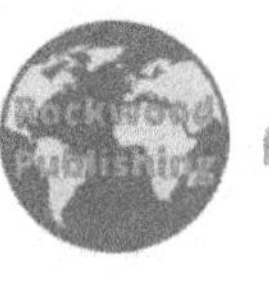
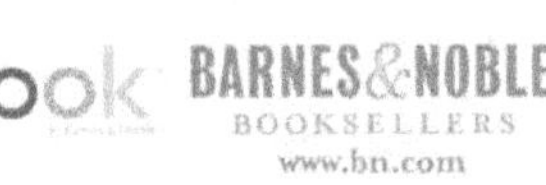

Disclaimers

The content contained within this book is for information and entertainment purposes only, and in no way purports to represent professional medical opinion. It should NOT be used as a substitute for expert advice, and you must consult with your designated health professional before acting upon any information contained herein or before undertaking any practice whose methodology is referred to in this book. The author is NOT a registered health professional and the text merely represents personal opinion, not medical fact. The author cannot be held responsible for the consequences of any action derived from the reading of this book, as the content is not based on diagnosis and subsequent regimen. It is the reader's responsibility to seek proper, professional medical advice from a registered health practitioner in connection with any material contained within this book.

Legal Disclaimer (part 1)

Nothing in this book should be construed as an attempt to diagnose, treat or cure. The information in this book is intended to be a community resource. The author takes no responsibility for any informational material or brochures produced using information taken from this book. The author has endeavoured to ensure that all information is correct at the time of publication. This information, however, is subject to change without notice. The author makes no warranty with regard to the accuracy of any

information and will not be liable for any errors or omissions. Any liability that arises as a result of this information is hereby excluded to the fullest extent allowed by law.
This information should not be used as a substitute for seeking independent professional advice.

Legal Disclaimer (part 2)

Disclaimer and Terms of Use:

a) i. In publishing this information, the author makes no representations concerning the efficacy, appropriateness or suitability of any products or treatments. Use this information at your own risk. The compiler is not a doctor and has no medical background or training.

ii. Statements and information regarding dietary supplements, books and any products mentioned have not been evaluated by any health authority and are not intended to diagnose, treat, cure or prevent any disease or health condition.

b) In view of the possibility of human error, neither the author nor any other party involved in providing this information, warrant that the information contained therein is in every respect accurate or complete and they are not responsible nor liable for any errors or omissions that may be found or for the results obtained from the use of such information. The entire risk as to use of this information is assumed by the user.

c) You are encouraged to consult other sources and confirm the information.

d) The information you access is provided "as is". No warranty, expressed or implied, is given as to the accuracy, completeness or timeliness of any information herein, or for obtaining legal advice. To the fullest extent permissible pursuant to applicable law, neither the author nor any other parties who have been involved in the creation, preparation, printing, or delivering of this information assume responsibility for the completeness, accuracy, timeliness, errors or omissions of said information and assume no liability for any direct, incidental, consequential, indirect, or punitive damages as well as any circumstance for any complication, injuries, side effects or other medical accidents to person or property arising from or in connection with the use or reliance upon any information contained herein.

e) The author is not responsible for the contents of any linked site or any link contained in a linked site, or any changes or update to such sites. The inclusion of any link does not imply endorsement by the author. The author makes no representations or claims as to the quality, content and accuracy of the information, services, products, messages which may be provided by such resources, and specifically disclaims any warranties, including but not limited to implied or express warranties of merchantability or fitness for any particular usage, application or purpose.

f) The information provided is general in nature and is intended for educational and informational purposes only. It is not intended to replace or substitute the evaluation, judgment, diagnosis, and medical or preventative care of a physician, paediatrician, therapist and/or health care provider.

g) Any medical, nutritional, dietetic, therapeutic or other decisions, dosages, treatments or drug regimes should be made in consultation with a health care practitioner. Do not discontinue treatment or medication without first consulting your physician, clinician or therapist.

h) By reading this information, you signify your assent to these terms and conditions of use. If you do not agree to these terms and conditions of use, do not read/use this information. If any provision of these terms and conditions of use shall be determined to be unlawful, void or for any reason unenforceable, then that provision shall be deemed severable from this agreement and shall not affect the validity and enforceability of any remaining provisions.

i) The information, services, products, messages and other materials, individually and collectively, are provided with the understanding that the author is not engaged in rendering medical advice or recommendations.

j) The information and the terms of use are subject to change without notice. The material provided as is without warranty of any kind and may include inaccuracies and/or typographical errors. The author makes no representations about the suitability of this information for any purpose. The author disclaims all warranties with regard to this information, including all implied warranties, and in no event shall the author be held liable, resulting from, or in any way related to, the use of this information.

k) The unauthorized alteration of the content of this information is expressly prohibited. The author, its agents and representatives shall not be responsible for any claims, actions or damages which may arise on account of the unauthorized alteration of this information.